Weight training
for Men

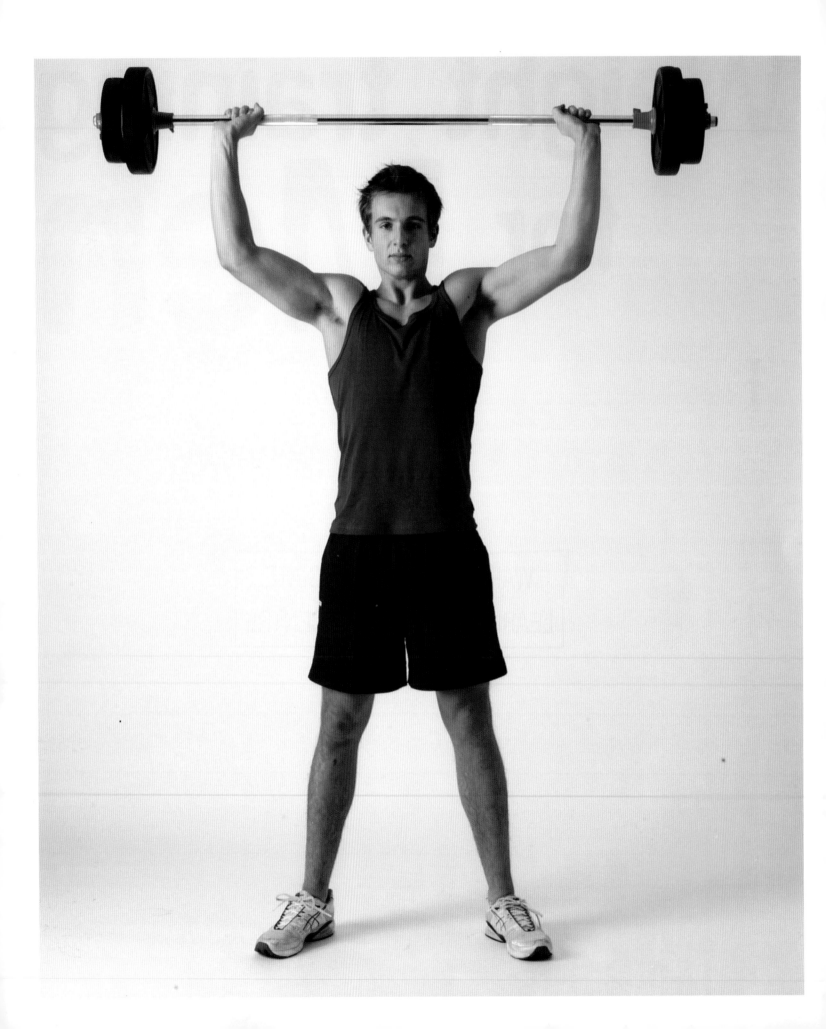

Weight training for Men

Grant Griffiths

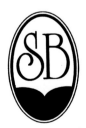

Published by SILVERDALE BOOKS
An imprint of Bookmart Ltd
Registered number 2372865
Trading as Bookmart Ltd
Desford Road
Enderby
Leicester LE19 4AD

© 2003 D&S Books Ltd

D&S Books Ltd
Kerswell,
Parkham Ash, Bideford
Devon, England
EX39 5PR

e-mail us at:-
enquiries@dsbooks.fsnet.co.uk

This edition printed 2003

Book code DS0066. Weight Training

ISBN 1-856057-76-3

Creative Director: Sarah King
Editor: Clare Haworth-Maden
Project editor: Sally MacEachern
Photographer: Colin Bowling
Designer: 2H Design

Typeset in Frutiger

Printed in China

1 3 5 7 9 10 8 6 4 2

Contents

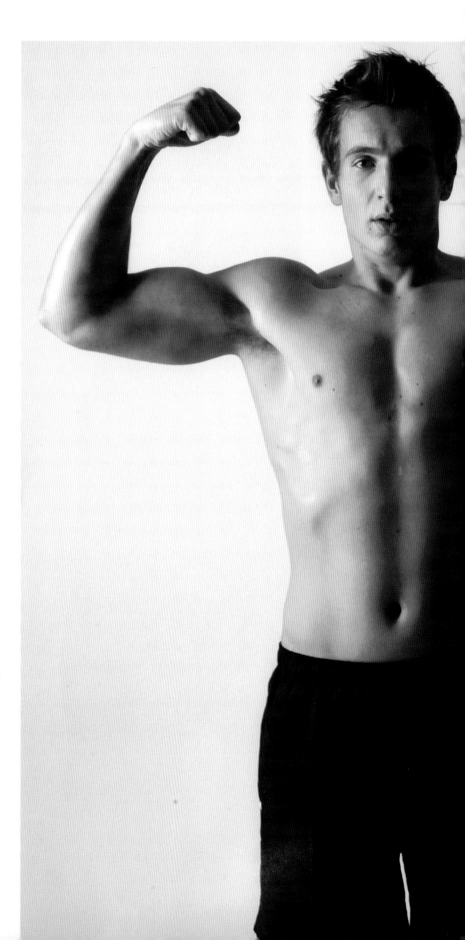

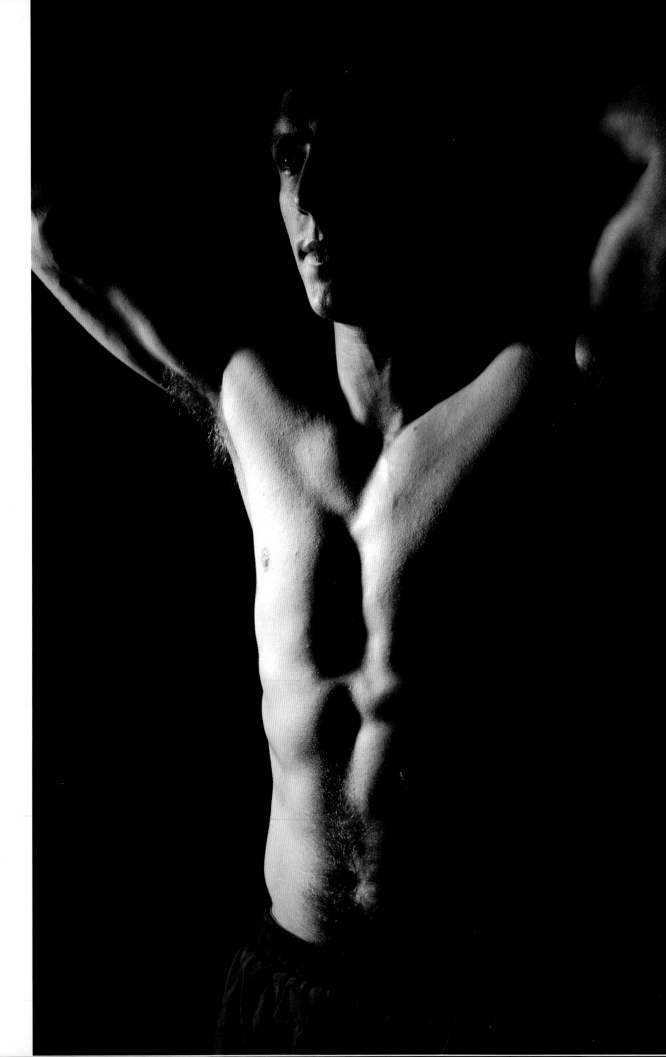

Introdution

The three stages of weight-training

If you are new to weight-training, you will need to work through the
beginner's stage before progressing through the intermediate to the
advanced stage. But regardless of whether you are
a beginner, intermediate or advanced weight-
trainer, always give your body a total workout.
Build, build, build is the key to success!

Tips for the beginner

So you're a beginner! You have made the decision to change your life
and your physique. The good news is that changing your diet and
starting an exercise programme will build bigger muscles quickly and relatively
easily, and all by performing one set of the exercises in this book. You will find
that the tips and guidelines included in this book will enable you to gain the
muscle mass you desire, without disrupting your normal life.

In general terms, you should lift about three times a week, keeping the weight
heavy enough to allow you to repeat any of the exercises six times.
Experimenting with the weight is the key to success. The important thing to
remember is that once you have built up to ten repetitions of each exercise, it
is then time to add weight and to drop back to the original six repetitions. I
call this the ten-repetition rule! If you do not do this, you will find that you are
allowing yourself to become stuck with the same old routine using the same
weight. This will not increase your muscle mass any further, but serves only to
sidetrack you into a dead end.

A variation of exercise, weight and, indeed, diet is the key to a
successful physical-development programme.

Tips for the intermediate trainer

As you may expect, when you reach the intermediate stage of weight-training, the routines
become a little more difficult. You should, by now, have started to see the physical results of
all of your hard work and dedication, so allow yourself some smug satisfaction at having
moved on in leaps and bounds. Now it's time to move on a little further.

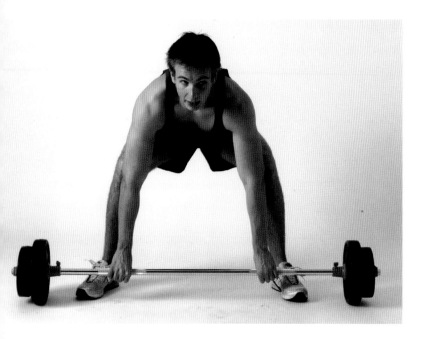

By now your body will require three sets of each exercise. It is still vitally important that you remember the rule of ten repeats that you learned when you were a beginner, however. At this intermediate stage of development, it is recommended that you perform each set of exercises as usual and also work with a suitable extra dumbbell or barbell weighted with a lighter weight.

After performing your usual set of exercises, repeat them using the lighter dumbbell or barbell until your muscles become exhausted and you literally cannot perform another repetition. This is called working your muscles to failure. You will feel that you have worked yourself really hard after this strenuous activity, and this regime is guaranteed to maximise muscle growth. When using this technique for development, it is always a good idea to work alongside a weight-training partner, someone who can help you if you get into any difficulties.

Tips for the advanced trainer

Congratulate yourself! You are now at the peak of your development and performance! You have learned the lessons of the intermediate stage of physical development very well. Now you will be using much more challenging poundage and will again follow the failure rule. Your routines will therefore be exhausting. Don't let this worry you, however, because you already have the muscle mass to overcome this demand and will really enjoy pushing your body in the gym.

When you reach this stage, you should have learned that your body is the best possible gauge of your performance. The key is to listen to what your body is telling you. And if you're feeling somewhat inadequate because you cannot lift as much as your training partner, it does not mean that your body is in any way weaker. Remember the characteristics of three basic body types, the endomorph, mesomorph and ectomorph (see page 20), and never allow yourself to become disheartened. There is no need to!

By now you will know the importance of piling on the weights. Never allow yourself to become stuck with, or complacent about, the same routines or patterns of activity. As was true for both previous stages of development, variety in exercise, weight and diet is the passport to success and maintenance.

Preparation

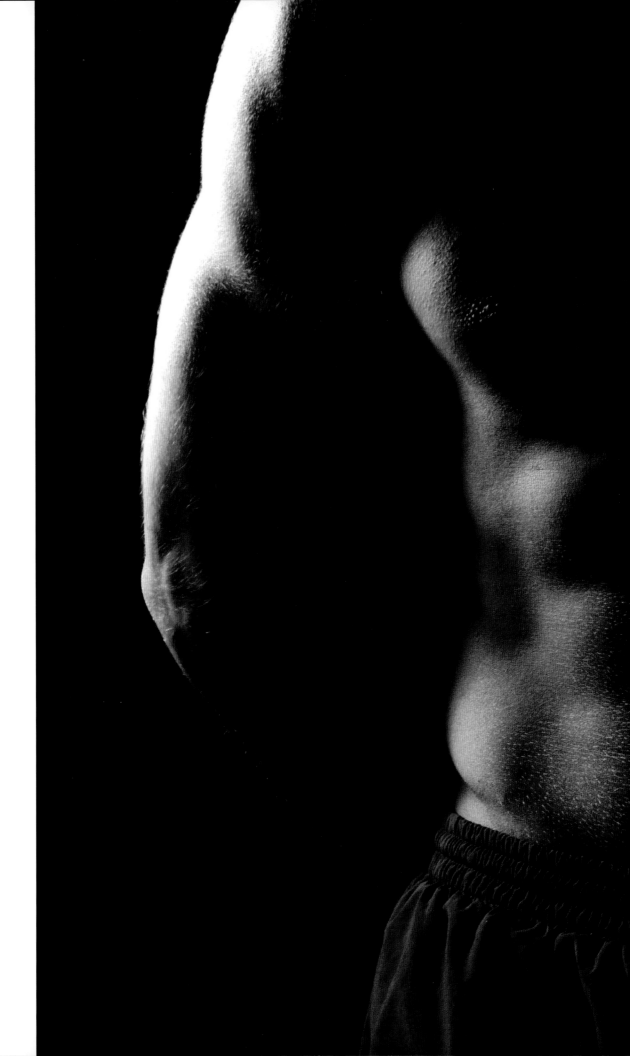

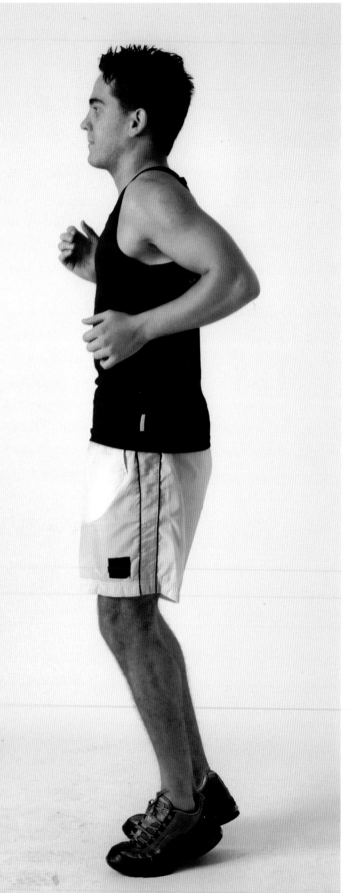

The warm-up

Before you embark on any serious exercise regime, it is vital to increase the blood supply to your muscle groups, as well as to build up some impetus for the exertions ahead. In other words, you will have to warm up! Starting with some light exercise will get your heart and lungs working harder, which will help your performance.

The best way to warm up your body is to perform some form of aerobic exercise (which does not mean bopping to loud music while bouncing around the room). A brisk walk, a light jog, swinging your arms or even climbing stairs will all help to pump blood into the muscle groups. Do any of the above for between five to ten minutes, and remember that this is only a warm-up to your exercise routine, not the routine itself.

Another activity that could have been designed as the perfect warm-up exercise is the press-up. If you can manage to do thirty press-ups in sequence, you will be ready for the more formal exercises that constitute your training regime.

Cooling down

After training, your muscles will be filled
with blood, and it is this that will give you
the feeling of being 'pumped'. Cooling
your body down after exercise is just as
important as priming it beforehand if you
are to achieve your physical goals, a simple
fact that is often ignored by those people
who concentrate only on actual strenuous
exercises.

Cooling down prevents the body's tissues
from retracting and tightening, thereby
warding off soreness and helping to
prevent injury. So always remember to do
some light aerobic activity for five minutes
before and after training. It will be five
minutes well spent, and you will definitely
feel the benefit afterwards.

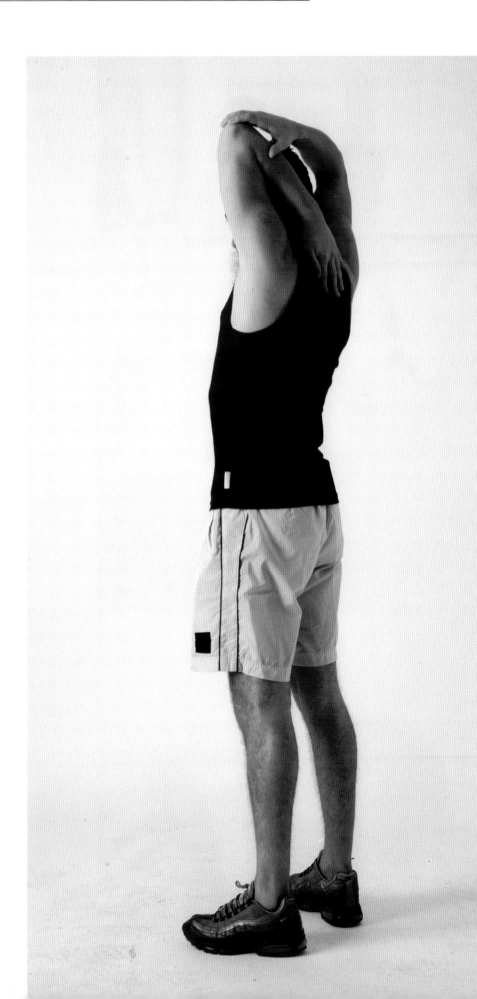

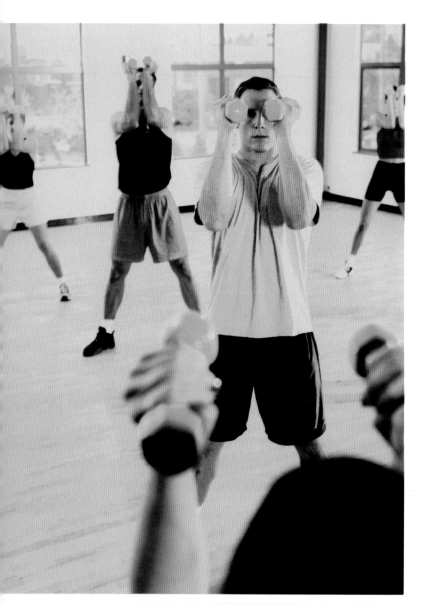

The equipment

The choice is yours as to whether to train at home or at a professional gym, but remember that using a commercial gym is rarely cheap (some of the more prestigious training facilities can cost upwards of a thousand pounds a year). One of the main selling points that gyms tend to promote is that they have all of the necessary expertise in house and can tailor an exercise programme to your requirements. Although this may be so, I can promise you that you will be forced play the waiting game. A workout that would normally take you one hour at home, for example, will often take twice as long in a commercial gym simply because other people will be queueing to use the equipment before you. And at peak times, the waiting period can be excessive.

The better, and cheaper, option is probably to purchase your own equipment. As your first expense, it is advisable to purchase 150kg (330lb) of weight, ranging from 10kg (22lb) to 0.25kg ($\frac{1}{2}$lb), a solid-milled bar, two solid-milled dumbbell bars and at least eight fast-released grips.

The exercise or weights bench comes in a number of forms and guises. Because individual body shapes and sizes can vary quite considerably, the best benchmark when testing one is actually to get on it and see if you feel comfortable. If you are in any doubt about your potential purchase, speak to a sales representative who is qualified to guide you. (This advice also applies to every single

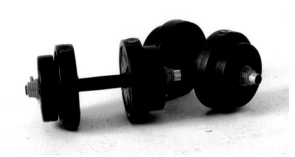

item of your weight-training equipment.) Always remember that quality is better than quantity, and the initial outlay on your purchase will hopefully give you an incentive to use it constructively to put you on the right track.

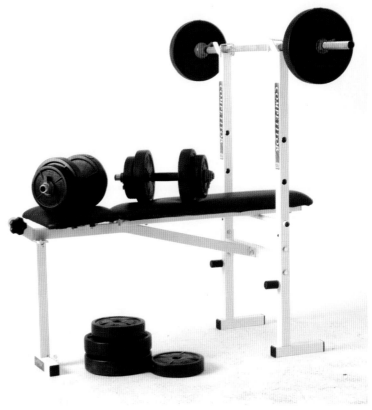

You will notice that certain specialist equipment is mentioned in several exercises in this book over and above the basic weights bench and weight discs. The ankle weight, for instance, is used to increase the physical resistance of your abdominal wall once your body has passed beyond the initial level of challenge, and is loaded with sand to provide this resistance. Care should be taken that ankle weights are always firmly, yet comfortably, secured. Another optional item that is required for certain exercises in this book is the chin bar, a piece of equipment that is relatively cheap and, in my opinion, worth buying. A solid-milled bar that fits within any solidly constructed doorframe, the chin bar is adjustable to match the width of any standard door. You must, however, take care to fit this item securely into solid wood, so that there is no possibility of movement. Remember that you should be the one who moves, not the chin bar or doorframe!

After your initial outlay, you could also purchase additional kilograms or pounds of weight as your training programme progresses.

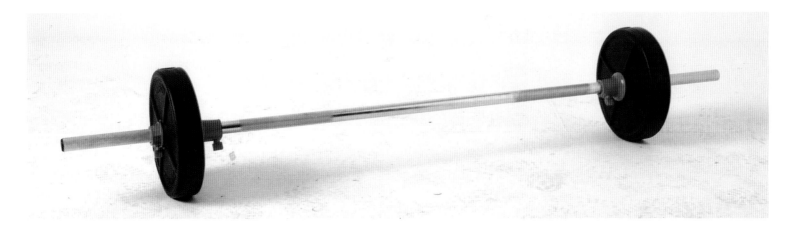

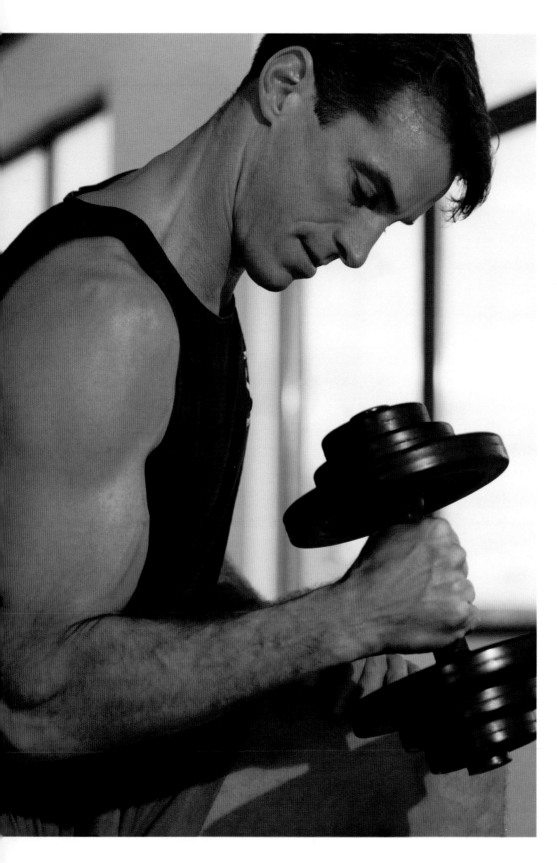

The right clothing for the job

When choosing the right apparel for exercise, common sense should be your watchword. You should definitely not wear a knitted or polo-neck jumper, for example, nor should you consider something loose that could catch on your equipment and increase the potential of injuring yourself or your partner. The important things to remember are that your clothing should neither be too tight nor too loose, but should still be comfortable and give you freedom of movement.

If you exercise in an environment that is normally quite cold, wearing sweatshirts or layers of clothing is a good idea because they can be removed as your exercise progresses and you warm up. Always remember to wear sensible footwear, such as training shoes, and *never* be so foolish as to exercise in bare feet in case you drop a 5kg (11lb) disc on your toes!

In fact, *always* be sensible and *never* fool around while weight-training. Treat your equipment and clothing with respect at all times, and remember that common sense rules!

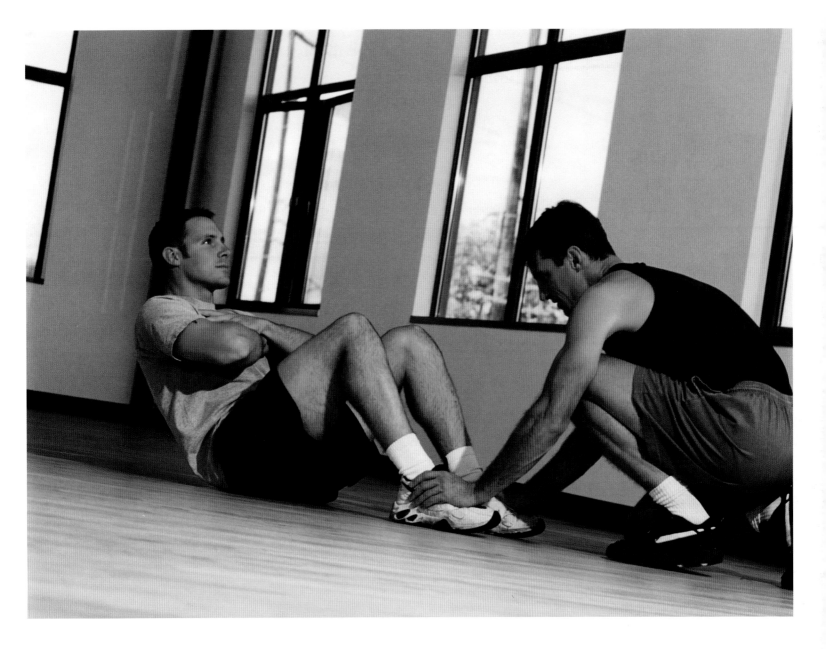

An exercise partner

Although you do not strictly need a training partner for every exercise in this book, from a safety point of view it is always a good idea to have someone around who could rescue you should you get into difficulties. This is particularly important when you are lifting heavy weights and find yourself in positions in which your muscles may fail. No matter how confident you may feel, a partner can quickly spot any signs of trouble, sometimes before you.

Apart from the safety angle, a partner is valuable in terms of motivation. If you exercise in company, you will find that you spur each other on to greater efforts.

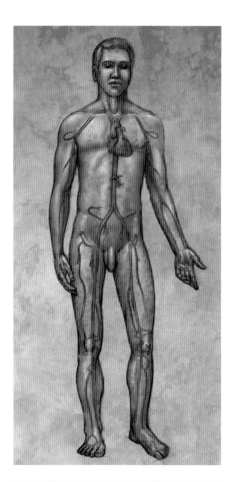

The body's muscular groups

To be technical, muscles comprise literally millions of tiny protein filaments that work together to produce motion in the body. We all possess more than six hundred individual muscles, which are served by nerves linking them to the spinal cord and brain.

Muscles are attached to the skeletal structure by tendons and other tissues. They work by exerting force, which converts chemical energy into the actions of tension and contraction. By simply contracting and becoming shorter in length, the movement of the muscles and muscular groups makes us capable of actions. To put it simply, muscles pull, but are incapable of pushing.

The basic needs of the body demand that muscles accomplish different tasks, which is why we are equipped with three distinct types of muscle. The cardiac muscles, which are found only in the heart, serve to pump blood around the body, but we are not concerned with the cardiac group of muscles in this book. The so-called 'smooth' muscles surround, cushion and protect our internal organs. These muscles do not require any exercise because they regulate themselves and operate by means of involuntary action, which is why the smooth muscles are also irrelevant to this book. The third, and most obvious, muscular group, consists of the muscles that we can exercise and develop. This is the skeletal muscle group, whose muscles can be consciously controlled.

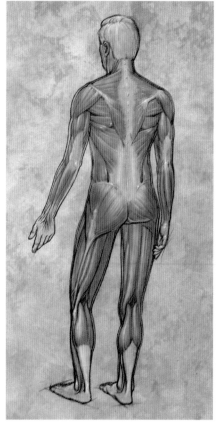

Male musculature.

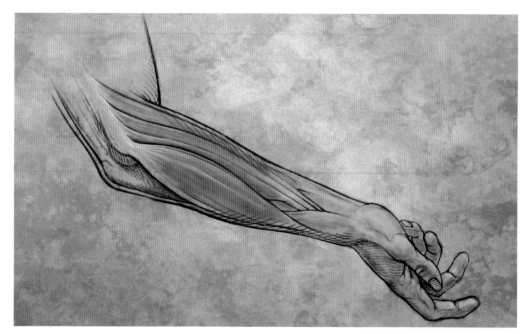

Muscles and tendons of the arm.

The skeletal muscles

In a man's body, the skeletal muscles make up approximately 40 per cent of his total weight. In a woman's body, these muscles comprise approximately 23 per cent of her total weight. We use these muscles for nearly every motion that the body makes, from flexing our fingers to walking, bending, stretching, running and, indeed, any other type of action that you can think of. Remember that muscles pull, but cannot push. In fact, muscles tend to pull equally from their attachments to the skeleton to their centres.

The skeletal muscles are also the most abundant type of muscular tissue. These are the muscles that we can see and feel, and that ache after strenuous exercise, but then, as they say, where there's no pain, there's no gain (see page 18). In order to develop these muscles, and therefore your body, into the form that you want, you will need dedication and a strong sense of purpose.

Because it is beyond the scope of this book to deal with all of the six hundred muscles in the human body, I have concentrated on some of the more obvious muscular groups for the purposes of physical development. There follows a rundown of these muscular groups, which will be dealt with more fully in section III: The exercises (see pages 41–110).

- The most prominent muscles of the shoulders are the deltoids.
- The arms possess muscles of the 'flexor' group. The upper arms are notable for the biceps. The lower arms have three main muscular groups, the brachiora dialis and the flexors and extensors that permit hand and wrist movement.
- The chest muscles consist of the pectoral major and the pectoral minor, collectively known as the pectorals or pecs. The pectoral major is a large muscle that joins the shoulder, collarbone and breastbone. The pectoral minor is located beneath this large muscle. The chest also possesses the clavicular upper, and sternal lower, chest fibres.
- The largest muscle in the back is the latissimus dorsi, usually referred to as the lats. Other muscular groups in the back are the rhomboids and the trapezius.
- The abdominal wall consists of the upper abs (abdominals), the lower abs and the lateral obliques.
- The largest muscle of the body is the gluteus maximus in the buttock area. Other muscles found in the buttocks are the gluteus medius and the gluteus minimus.
- The four large muscles in the thighs are called the quadrilaterals or quads. The hamstrings are also found here, which consist of three muscular groups at the back of the thigh.
- Finally, the calf muscles are technically known as the gastrocnemius, the tibialis anterior and the soleus.

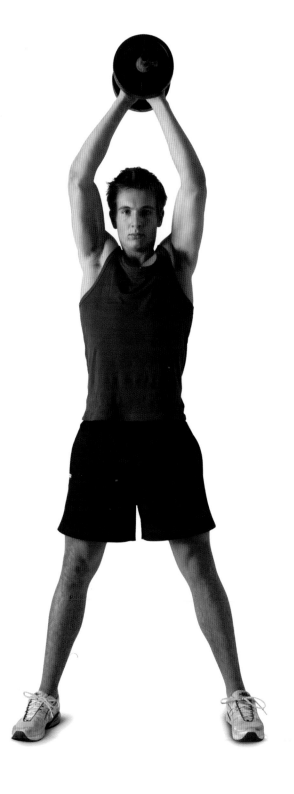

No pain, no gain!

Many people think that pain is a bad thing, often with good reason! In terms of weight-training, a certain amount of pain is, however, a good thing.

Pain is the body's way of telling you that you should rest and that you have worked a certain muscle part to its full potential. It's therefore important to remember that even though your exercise regime is vital to your physical development, resting your muscles sufficiently is equally, if not more, important because when your muscles have been worked particularly hard, they will inevitably be torn and damaged. This is part of the body's natural process of building and repairing and is nothing to worry about.

Remember that muscle growth will not be achieved without sufficient rest because it is during periods of rest that the muscles repair themselves and grow.

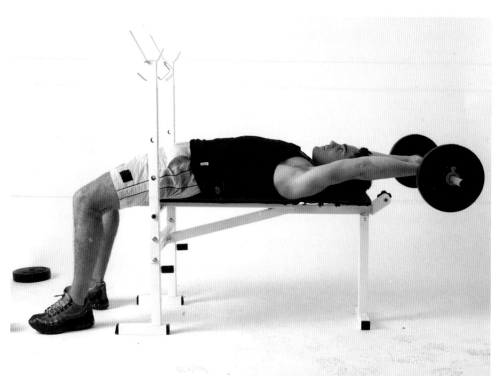

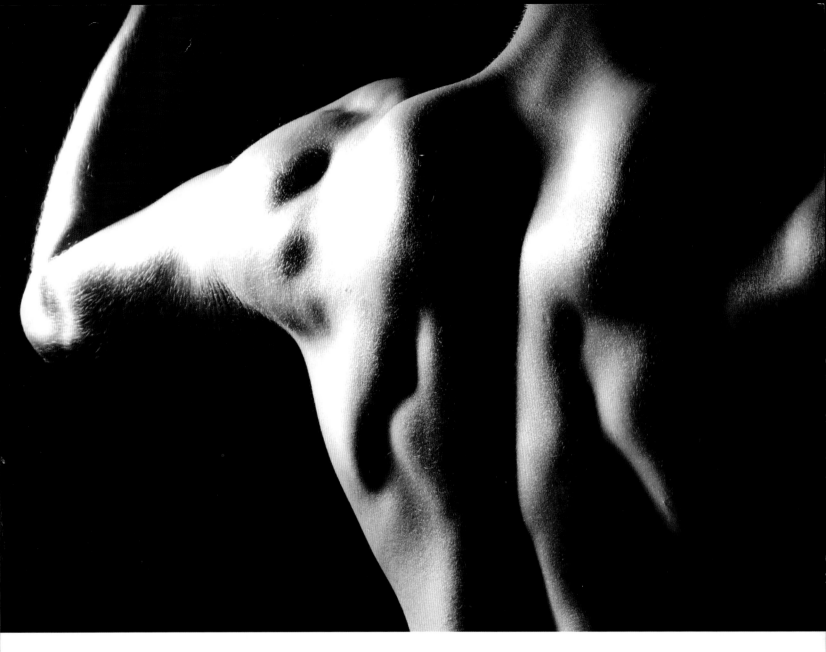

Nutrition

Many people who have had the personal dedication to embark on a weight-training programme are surprised when the results of their efforts are minimal. Although they may be pumping all the iron that they can lift, this is often because they have neglected the most important factor, the vital ingredient being a sensible approach to nutrition.

For a weight-training regime to be successful, a well-balanced diet is a basic requirement. In my personal experience, I have observed people struggle to gain muscle mass while on a faddish diet based on a solitary dietary factor. The strenuous effort – efforts that are otherwise admirable – of those who rely solely on a diet of either carbohydrates or protein are doomed to failure.

But before looking at the basics of sensible nutrition, we must first consider the subject of body shape.

Body profiles

Genetically speaking, there are three types of body shape, ranging from the heavily overweight, through the athletically proportioned, to the skinny. These types are technically described as endomorphic, mesomorphic and ectomorphic. You will inevitably fall into one of these categories, but whatever shape you naturally happen to be, it is important to realise that sensible nutrition, combined with a suitable training programme, will cause you to gain significant muscle mass.

Most people are a combination of these three basic types, and determining which you most closely resemble will give you an idea of how muscular you will end up looking, regardless of how hard you work out.

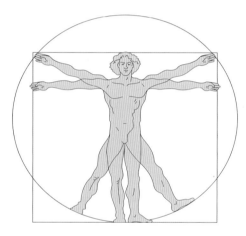

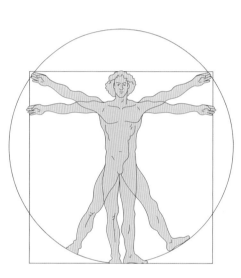

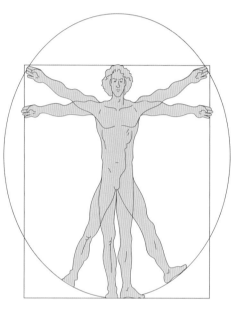

The endomorph

The predominant factor in the endomorphic body form is a propensity to gain weight. People of this type are generally rounded and short in stature and tend to have more fat cells than people of the other two groups. If you happen to be an endomorph, you have luck on your side, however: because your body readily puts on weight, it provides you with a ready-made fuel reserve to help you to lay down muscle.

The mesomorph

An easy way to spot a mesomorphic body shape is to look at any athlete, the advantages of this body type having usually ensured that he or she became an athlete in the first place. Mesomorphs are naturally muscular, with wide shoulders, slim waists, minimal body fat and an obviously defined frame. People of this type can eat large amounts and find it relatively easy to put on weight. In addition, the mesomorph usually has no difficulty in gaining extra muscle mass.

The ectomorph

The frame of the ectomorphic type is easy to spot: generally long and thin, ectomorphs often possess wiry strength, but have minimal reserves of muscle and fat. In the terminology of weight-training, the ectomorph is often described as being a 'hard-gainer' because it is believed that this type finds it difficult to lay down fat and muscle reserves. If you are an ectomorph, don't be disheartened, however, because this minor problem can be overcome with a sensible diet plan.

Nutrition without suffering

Having decided on your body type, you can now plan a nutritional programme that is suitable for your physical shape and size, without subjecting yourself to unnecessary hardship.

Unlike most diets, which are usually designed for weight loss and are therefore very restrictive, here's the good news: a weight-training diet lets you eat six or seven times a day! Having said that, this doesn't mean that you can gorge yourself on a mound of burgers and fries, an approach that would only succeed in increasing your waist size rather than improving your physique. Little and often should be your motto. Remember, too, that the thing to avoid is the stomach rumble because feeling hungry is a sure indication that you are burning up precious reserves of fuel, fuel that you need to build muscle! This body fuel is expressed in terms of calories (put simply, a calorie is a unit of energy.)

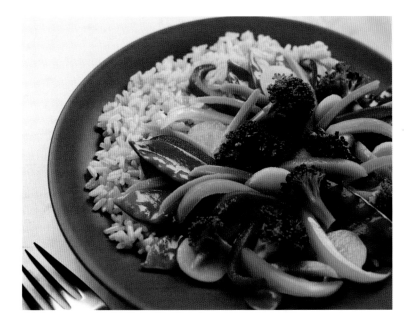

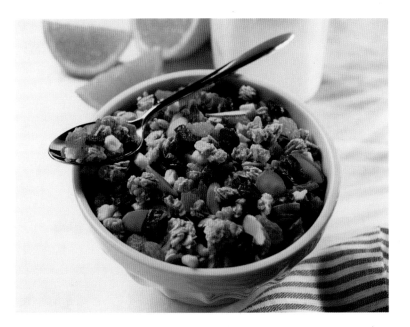

This rule is even more important if your body shape is ectomorphic, when the six-or-seven-meals-a-day plan can actually be increased by a further 600 calories per day. Some people have all the luck!

It is an eating plan whose sole purpose is to maintain your fuel reserves (calories) at a constant level. To this end, the 'little and often' rule applies at all times. If you gorge yourself at one sitting, all that you will achieve in the aftermath of your feast is flushing all of the beneficial calories out of your system. Having smaller, more frequent, meals will, on the other hand, vastly increase your muscle-building potential. Ignore this basic rule of weight-training, and you can pump iron for twenty-four hours a day, seven days a week, but it will not make a bit of difference to the state of your physique. Sensible nutrition, combined with a sensible weight-training programme, is the key to successful muscle gain.

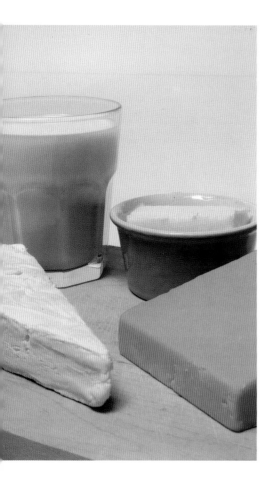

Protein

Protein is the basic building block required to lay down muscle. It is found in large quantities in meat products, such as chicken, fish, beef and pork, and also forms a major component of dairy products and nuts.

Protein is called a 'quick-fix' food because it delivers a sudden burst of energy rather than a steadily released amount. Your body will burn off this injection of energy very quickly, usually within an hour or so. Remember, however, that a steady release of energy is preferable and that you must prevent your stomach from rumbling with hunger.

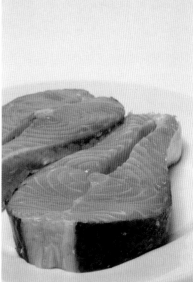

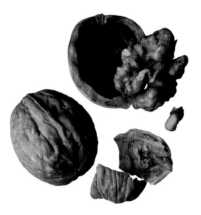

The importance of protein

When you have settled into your own weight-lifting routine, tiny muscular tears are inevitable because you are using your muscle groups far more vigorously than you did previously. This is not a big problem because the body uses the protein in your diet not only to repair, but also to build up, the muscles, making them stronger and larger. Remember to derive your protein from healthy animal or plant-food products, such as lean chicken, tuna, beef, nuts and grains.

Because it cannot make you a muscle man on its own, protein must be combined with the other two food groups (carbohydrates and fats). Loading your body with protein alone will also hurt your body rather than help it because excess protein is stored in the body as fat – the last thing you want.

Carbohydrates

This weight-training diet plan is based on carbohydrates because carbohydrates are more easily converted into energy than protein within the body

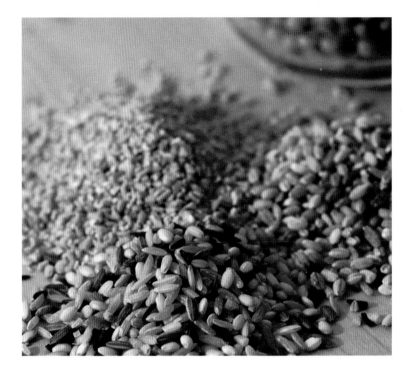

Carbohydrates are found in 'bulky' foods that are considered to be 'fillers', generally wheat- and grain-based products, such as bread, pasta, cereals and also potatoes and fruit.

Carbohydrates deliver a slow, constant supply of energy over a long period of time. This means that the carbohydrate group in your diet should provide the basic fuel for your day-to-day life, thereby freeing up the energy provided by protein for muscle build-up and repair.

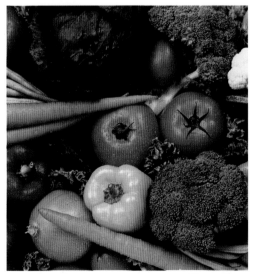

'Good' fats and 'bad' fats

Although many people seem to be convinced that protein alone is the key to successful muscle gain, they couldn't be further from the truth! A diet that consists solely of nuts, tuna, chicken or beefsteak will not help in any way. To ensure success, the protein must be balanced with carbohydrates and *fats*!

While we are on the subject of fat, it is commonly thought that fat is bad for you. This belief, like many others, is a complete myth, however. An average man whose diet consists of 2,000 calories a day actually needs 90g (about 3oz) of fat for his body to function properly. On average, a woman will consume 1,200 calories a day and will need a minimum of 65g (about 2oz) of fat.

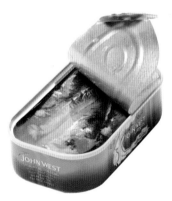

The truth of the matter is that there are considerable differences between types of fat. In short, there are 'good' fats and 'bad' fats. The 'good' fats, which are called polyunsaturated fats, are found in fish, vegetables and nuts, and in also in olive oil and grain-based products. A healthy rule to follow is that the majority of your fat intake should come from plant sources rather than meat products.

The bad boys are the saturated fats, of which there are many. Saturated fats are very, very bad for you because they clog up the arteries and cause the wrong sort of weight gain. These fats are found in sausages, burgers and highly processed meat products. The easiest way to tell the 'good' from the 'bad' fats is that the beneficial, polyunsaturated fats, like vegetable oil, are liquid at room temperature, while the harmful, saturated fats, such as lard and butter, are solid.

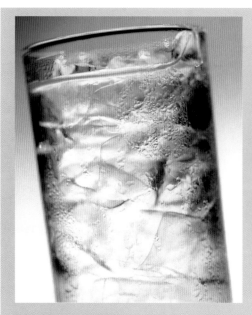

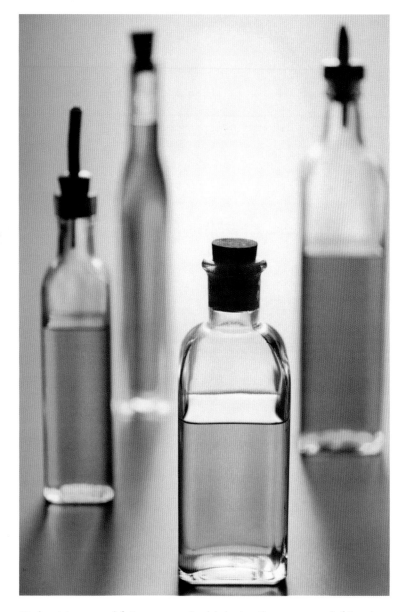

Liquid intake

Consuming a lot of watery drinks should be an important part of your nutritional regime. Weight-trainers cannot perform to their optimum potential unless they do. It is especially important to drink large amounts of water (or other appropriate beverages, such as sports drinks) before, during and after exercising. This will aid rehydration, flood your bloodstream with carbohydrates and shorten your body's recovery time.

The first fuel stop

People who weight-train before breakfast, the first fuel stop of the day, aren't doing themselves or their energy levels any favours! Having been fasting all night, their body has slowed down and is subsisting on last night's evening meal. All of the body's rations are low before breakfast, and there's a particular shortfall in the blood's glucose and glycogen levels.

It's therefore not advisable to work out before you have consumed enough calories to raise your energy levels to an acceptable rate. The best way of receiving a quick calorie boost and kick-starting your system is to eat fruit, yoghurt, toast or a good-quality sports drink. Never, ever train on an empty stomach!

It's best to regard fat as a good, old, but rather wayward, friend, one whose company you enjoy, but has the habit of getting you into trouble. It's fine to let it into your life in small doses at particular times, but too much, or too little, are both damaging. (If you cut fat out of your diet entirely, you will not gain weight, but will instead end up looking like a stick insect.) The key to dealing with it is not to develop a fat phobia, but to treat it like any other component of your diet: enjoy it in moderation, little and often and always as part of a well-balanced diet plan.

Matching your diet plan to your body type

Before we look at the three diet plans, remember that they should be based on carbohydrates and fats to enable your body to utilise the slow release of energy that they supply in order to free up protein to build and repair muscle tissue.

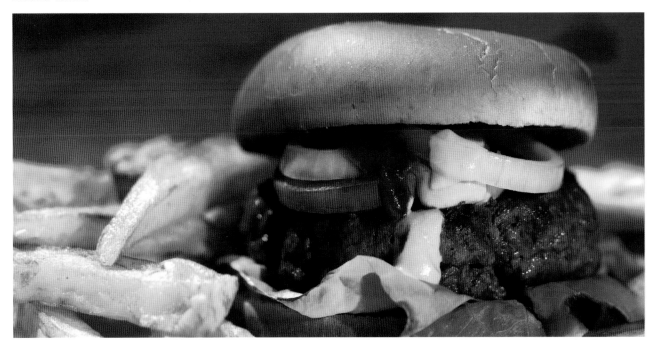

Calorie-packed snacks and breakfasts should not be indulged in too frequently by endomorphs.

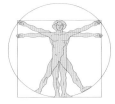

The endomorphic diet

Just to remind you: the endomorph is a large person who needs to shed some weight. It is important to realise that your body shape is not bad! In fact, the endomorphic body shape has a lot of advantages, not least the ability to gain weight easily. The trick is to gain muscle mass rather than fatty tissue, which is why the saturated fats found in chips, doughnuts, sweets and all of the foods that we love so much, but know are bad for us are – you've guessed it – a definite no-no! (But if you can't cut them out of your diet, at least try to reduce your consumption of them dramatically.)

The bad news

The trouble with being an endomorph is that you have an appetite to match your size. It therefore wouldn't be surprising if you raided the fridge and kitchen cupboards in the dead of night, and then awoke in the morning and repeated the exercise by demolishing a fully cooked breakfast loaded with saturated fats, with the rest of the day being punctuated with calorie-packed snacks between calorie-loaded meals. You don't need me to tell you that these habits are destructive, both to your health and your training approach.

That's enough of the bad news! Let's take the positive approach and deal with your daily diet step by step, as well as improving your state of mind about yourself, increasing your confidence and improving your physical frame.

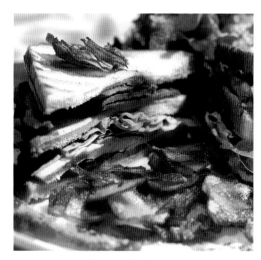

A cooked breakfast is fine for endomorphs as long as you avoid frying food.

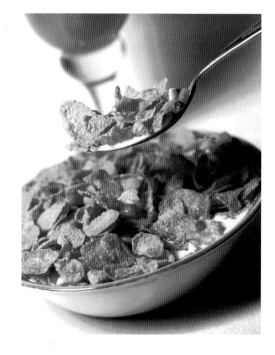

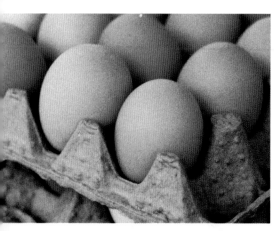

Breakfast: the good news

Breakfast is important! Not only is it sensible to eat a good breakfast when weight-training, it should, in fact, be the first of your 'little and often' meals.

The really good news is that you can start the day with a fully cooked breakfast consisting of sausages, bacon, bread, tomatoes, mushrooms and eggs, as long as it is prepared in the right way. Rather than frying, this means grilling or poaching and removing any visible fat, such as bacon rind. Try to cut out the frying process completely or, at the very least, reduce it to the bare minimum, and even then, always use a vegetable-based cooking oil. You now have a fully cooked breakfast with the guilt removed, so enjoy it!

The same message applies to all of your other meals and snacks: lean is the key! Remember that the basic rule of little and often applies as much to you as it does to the skinniest ectomorph.

Here are a few cereal- and egg-based ideas with which to vary your breakfast experience.

Cereals

Flake-based cereals like bran, corn or rice products are a good way of obtaining vitamins and minerals after fasting throughout the night. Avoid those flakes to which a sugar frosting has been added, however (it's healthier to add any sweetening yourself).

A breakfast of cereal combined with semi-skimmed milk (not skimmed, which tastes vile), such fruits as bananas, pears, peaches, grapefruits or oranges (any of which can also be taken in the form of juice), plus two slices of toast (frugally spread with butter or margarine and maybe a preserve), will sustain your dietary needs until mid-morning.

Eggs

The egg is the perfect nutritional hit! That small shell actually contains everything that your body needs. Combine a poached, scrambled or boiled egg with a slice of toast (spread with a small amount of butter or margarine and perhaps a preserve) and a piece of fruit, and you have a naturally well-balanced breakfast. If you are attempting to lose weight and want to tuck into more than one egg, remove one or two yokes and eat only the whites. (The yoke contains cholesterol, while the white is pure protein.)

Midday meals

Meals eaten at midday should ideally consist of vegetables, protein and carbohydrates, so if you usually consume pies, chips, pastries and pizza, they're out, I'm afraid.

Always plan ahead: you should put as much planning into your midday meals as you do into breakfast. It is a good idea to vary your diet on a daily basis to avoid boredom, so take the trouble to draw up a detailed weekly diet sheet and then stick to it. As an endomorph, you already know how hard it is to stick to your good intentions, but if you make the effort, the results will be worth it.

Here are a few suggestions for midday meals that will fulfil your dietary needs, as well as defeating lunchtime boredom.

- Team a tuna or chicken sandwich or baguette with as much salad as you can eat. The only danger area to avoid here is drenching your salad with gallons of dressing or mayonnaise. Always choose a healthy dressing, and go for a low-fat product every time (there's not much difference in taste anyway). This option is particularly suitable if you are at work.

- If you have more time on your hands and can prepare a meal at home, opt for pasta, fruit and wholemeal bread. With this meal, as with all others, a sensible combination of the three food groups – protein, carbohydrates and polyunsaturated fats – is the key to reducing your body fat and increasing your muscle-gaining potential.

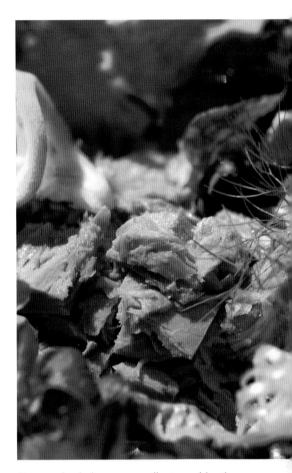

Tuna and salad are an excellent combination – just remember to keep dressings low-fat.

Evening meals

Correct timing is the key to your evening meals. It is not advisable to eat after 8pm due to the way your body functions. If you eat late, it will be uncomfortably close to bedtime, and sleeping after a heavy meal will tempt your body to utilise the calories that you have consumed for laying down fat, so try not to go to bed on a full stomach. I have found that the optimum time for an evening meal is between 7 and 8pm because eating at this time gives your body the chance to process the nutrients that it has received in a productive way.

It is very important to plan your meals in advance and to ensure that you always have the right ingredients to hand with which to make a healthy meal. If you do not, temptation can take over and lead you into making a mistake, thereby undoing all the good that you have done throughout the day.

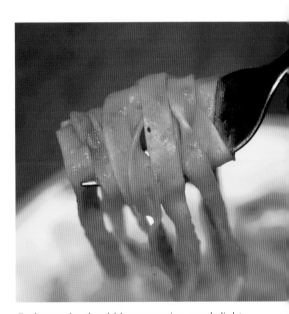

Endomorphs should keep evening meals light – and make sure you eat early in the evening.

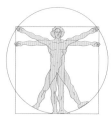

The mesomorphic diet

Just to jog your memory: the mesomorph is an athletic person who is naturally muscular. Although mesomorphs are already ahead in the weight-training game, don't let your natural advantages go to your head and become careless about your diet. Taking care of your diet is, in fact, as important a factor in your training plan as it is for endomorphic and ectomorphic types. Like endomorphs, the trick for mesomorphs is to gain muscle mass rather than fatty tissue, and even though you don't have to be quite so careful about reducing the amount of fat in your diet, it's still inadvisable to allow your arteries to become furred up by consuming too many saturated fats.

Taking a positive approach to your daily diet is vital if you are to maintain both your health and your physique. Just because you can eat chocolate and chips without piling on the kilos does not mean that you should. And remember that although mesomorphs may be athletic when they are young, their frame has a tendency to become more endomorphic in middle age. A well-balanced diet will, however, help to ward off this problem.

The bad news

The trouble with being a mesomorph is that although you can eat anything with no apparent ill effects, there are, unfortunately, negative consequences, even if you aren't aware of them. Like the endomorph, you, too, are likely to raid the fridge in the wee, small hours and then start the day by demolishing a fully cooked breakfast loaded with saturated fats, while the rest of the day could be punctuated with calorie-packed snacks between calorie-laden meals. These habits are destructive to your health.

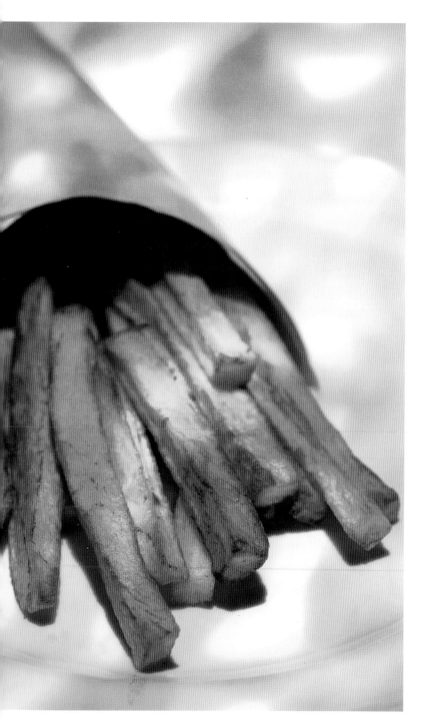

Just because mesomorphs can eat some fatty foods does not mean they should indulge too often.

Breakfast: the good news

The good news for mesomorphs is that you are naturally muscular, and that the food that you consume is fast-tracked to the musculature. You can't go wrong if you stick to the 'little and often' rule, starting with a healthy, well-balanced breakfast and then spreading your food intake throughout the rest of the day.

Like endomorphs, you can start the day with a fully cooked breakfast comprising bacon, sausages, eggs, tomatoes, mushrooms, bread and all of the trimmings, as long as you grill or poach it and remove any visible fat, including bacon rind. Try to avoid the frying process completely, or at least to fry food as little as possible and, when you do, always use a vegetable-based cooking oil. This will result in a 'ripped', or very defined, body type.

Alternatively, here are some ideas for cereal- or egg-based breakfasts.

Cereals

As far as cereals are concerned, the advice given on page 26 for the endomorphic type applies just as much to you.

Eggs

A good way of meeting your body's nutritional requirements after a night's sleep is to have an egg, whose shell contains everything that your body needs. Teaming a poached, scrambled or boiled egg with a slice of toast (spread with a little butter or margarine and perhaps a preserve) and a piece of fruit will give you a well-balanced breakfast. A healthy way of enjoying the nutrients that two eggs offer is to scramble them (the yokes, as well as the whites) with a small amount of vegetable oil and semi-skimmed milk. If you crave a fried egg (and you, along with ectomorphs, can usually get away with it), make sure that you fry it in a tiny amount of polyunsaturated oil.

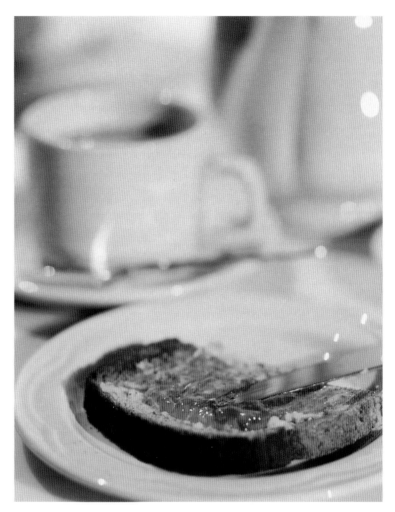

Mesomorphs should start the day with a light, healthy breakfast.

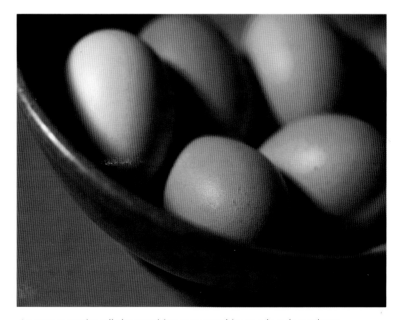

An egg contains all the nutrition you need in one handy package.

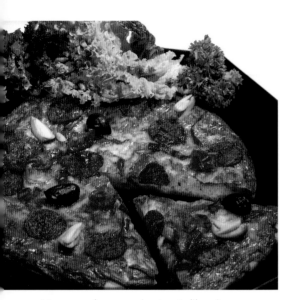

Mesomorphs can enjoy treats like pizza on occasion.

Midday meals

At the risk of sounding repetitive, mesomorphs can get away with eating all sorts of goodies, but that doesn't necessarily mean that you should! Although you have far more leeway in terms of your eating habits than the endomorphic type, it is still advisable to plan your meals in advance and not to eat on the run. Take the time to plan a sensible diet plan on a weekly basis, ensuring that you vary your meals to combat boredom. Pay particular attention to including the three food groups (protein, carbohydrates and fats) in your diet, and place special emphasis on reducing your intake of saturated fats to the barest minimum.

Here are some suggestions to help you to vary your lunchtime diet.

• A hot or cold pasta, tuna or chicken salad provides a balance of the three food groups. If you can, supplement this dish with some fruit or vegetables. The advantage of this type of meal is that it can be prepared in advance, stored in Tupperware containers and taken wherever you are going so that you never have to miss a meal (always bear in mind the 'little and often' rule).

• Fancy a pizza? Yes, you read it correctly, pizza! Two slices, in fact! Pizza admittedly contains some 'bad', saturated fats, but then you are a mesomorph and can get away with the occasional lapse. If any endomorphs are reading this section, pizza remains forbidden to you, unless it is a low-fat product, and the low-fat option is, of course, best for mesomorphs, too. And always remember to try to combine whatever you are eating with fruit, salad or vegetables.

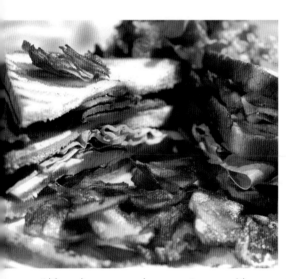

Although mesomorphs can get away with some dietary lapses, early, healthy meals are best.

Evening meals

All of the advice given to mesomorphs for breakfast and midday meals applies to evening meals as well. Because it is not a good idea to go to bed feeling too full, the optimum time to eat is usually between 7 and 8pm.

Remember that it is important to plan your meals in advance and to ensure that you always have the ingredients to hand with which to make a healthy meal. Although you can often get away with proverbial murder in your diet, temptation may gain the upper hand if you don't plan ahead, leading you to sin by indulging in such junk food as burgers, pies and chips.

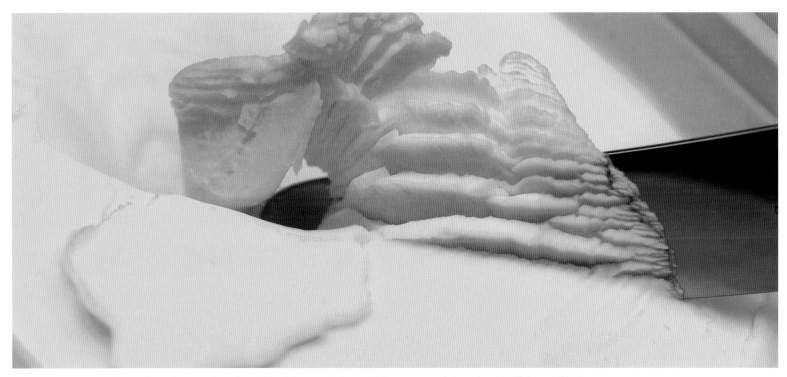

Although ectomorphs can largely eat what they like without gaining weight, saturated fats should still be avoided.

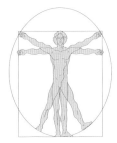

The ectomorphic diet

Ectomorphs are generally slim and are described as 'hard-gainers' because they may have difficulty gaining solid muscle mass. This is why the ectomorphic type can eat relatively vast amounts of food without putting on weight. Although some would regard this as an advantage, it is not conducive to muscle gain, but there are ways around this problem.

The 'little and often' rule applies even more to ectomorphs than to the other two body types. And unlike endomorphs and mesomorphs, you can safely add 600 extra calories to your diet per day.

Taking a positive approach and dealing with your daily diet step by step should improve your self-perception, your confidence and your physical frame.

The bad news

The problem with being an ectomorph is that you can eat anything you like, but put on little or no weight, weight that many ectomorphs desperately want to gain. Raiding the fridge in the middle of the night will make no difference to this type, especially if it is part of a 'binge'. (Binge-eating is the great failing of the ectomorph, not least because it is not conducive to muscle gain.) Sticking to the 'little and often' rule is essential for this type. Finally, saturated fats are just as bad for the slim ectomorph as they are for endomorphs and mesomorphs.

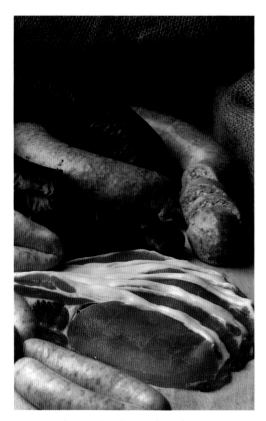

Ectomorphs need to begin their day with a hearty breakfast – but remember to avoid frying food.

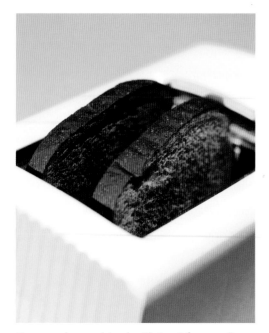

Eggs can be combined with toast for a well-balanced breakfast.

Breakfast: the good news

Ectomorphs can safely eat more for breakfast than the other two body types. It is, however, important that they eat strategically, possibly by making up a shake supplement (see page 39) in the morning and sipping it with food throughout the day, to give their bodies the extra 600 sustaining calories that they require daily.

Ectomorphs often have difficulty eating early in the morning and can fall into the habit of drinking copious amounts of beverages like tea or coffee, which is bad news because it tends to keep the body in 'starvation mode'. Ectomorphs should therefore make a real effort to kick-start their systems in the morning with a hearty breakfast. The really good news is that ectomorphic types needn't concern themselves with the amount that they eat. In fact, the more food, the better. Bearing that in mind, it is not so much a case of 'little and often' as 'a little more and often!'

It is still important for ectomorphs to cut saturated fats from their diet. So even though it is good to begin your day with a fully cooked breakfast consisting of sausages, bacon, bread, tomatoes, mushrooms and eggs, grilling or poaching your food is a far better option than frying it. It is also advisable to remove any visible fat, such as the rind from bacon. In fact, try not to fry any food at all, but if you occasionally must, use only vegetable-based oils.

To sum up, with the exception of saturated fats, ectomorphs should always add food to their meals, never take it away!

Cereals

Apart from increasing the amount of cereals eaten in combination with fruit and full-fat milk, the advice given to endomorphs (see page 26) applies to ectomorphs as well.

Eggs

The egg can be compared to a large vitamin pill; as a nutritional hit, it is hard to beat! When a poached, scrambled or boiled egg is combined with a slice of toast spread with butter or margarine, and perhaps a preserve, and a piece of fruit, it provides a well-balanced breakfast. Scrambled eggs make a good start to the day for ectomorphs, and perhaps you should consider having three eggs to help you to give your body the extra 600 calories that it needs a day. Prepare three whole eggs (yokes and whites) with a small amount of vegetable oil and full-fat milk and then scramble away. If you'd prefer a fried egg (ectomorphs and mesomorphs can get away with it), have two, but make sure that you fry them in a very small amount of polyunsaturated oil.

Midday meals

Because people of the ectomorphic type can eat more than anyone else, no meal should present a particular problem, that is, as long as you keep the balance of the three food groups (protein, carbohydrates and fat) in the right proportion. Like mesomorphs and endomorphs, you should include some fruit, salad or vegetables in every meal, lunch included.

If you are taking a shake supplement, you could have a portion of this with your midday meal rather than downing it all in one go. And although I've referred to a midday meal, it could actually be several small meals spaced out throughout the day, which is the best option for your physical type.

Although, like mesomorphs, you can get away with eating just about anything, and as slim as you are, it's still advisable to reduce your intake of saturated fats. You may want to gain weight, but this weight should be in the form of muscle mass, not fat reserves.

Try the following lunchtime ideas.

- A lean-turkey and sausage sandwich crammed with lettuce, tomatoes and, indeed, anything else that you can squeeze between two slices of bread. Better still, have two lean-turkey and sausage sandwiches!
- Fruit should put in a lunchtime appearance as dessert.
- In addition, have a natural yoghurt, as well as your supplementary shake, to add much-needed extra calories to your diet.

If you find it difficult to eat this much at one sitting, don't have one meal, but several, spaced out throughout the day (and sip your shake rather than gulping it down). In fact, ectomorphs will find spacing out their food intake far more comfortable and beneficial than consuming one huge meal.

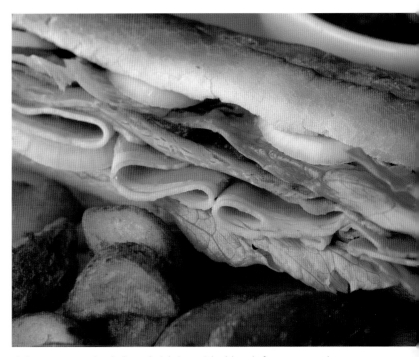

A lean meat and salad sandwich is an ideal lunch for ectomorphs.

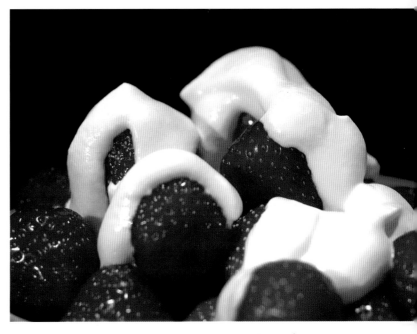

Make sure you eat fruit – supplemented with yoghurt – for extra calories.

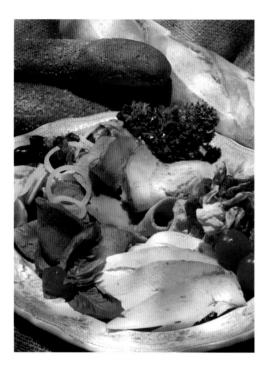

Evening meals

As far as food intake is concerned, ectomorphs again come out best in the evening-meal stakes. Just remember that you are trying to lay down muscle, not fat, so that consuming 500g of chocolate instead of a healthy, well-balanced meal is not going to get you anywhere. I know that you are always on the go, but try to slow down while you are eating, and afterwards, to give your body the chance to absorb the nutrients from your food. If, like many ectomorphs, you find the process of eating boring, the following psychological trick may help: don't pile your food onto one large plate, but instead think 'buffet' and divide it between several small dishes.

It's also advisable to eat before 8pm and never to go to bed feeling full, otherwise your body may 'waste' the nutrients that you have given it, so undoing all of your good work.

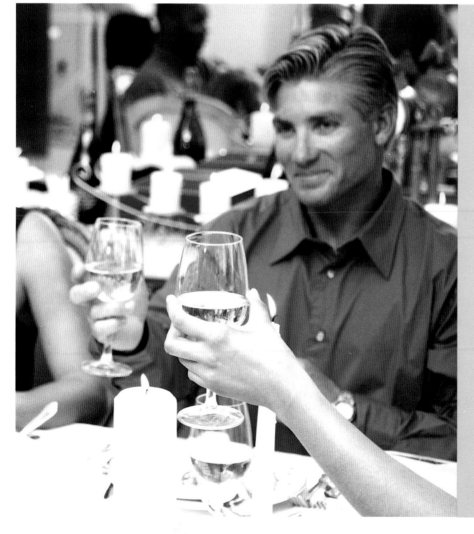

Eating out

There are few times when temptation is more difficult to resist than when one is eating out. If all of your good intentions tend to fly out of the window in a restaurant, you may not understand how the food you are eating is prepared or how much fat it contains. So here are a few helpful tips to bear in mind when looking at a menu.

- Avoid any dish that the menu states is fried, breaded, crispy, scampi-style, creamed, *au gratin* or served with gravy because it will be loaded with fat.
- Choose dishes that are described as being broiled, charbroiled, poached, prepared in their own juices, cooked in a tomato sauce or marinated. These options should provide enough variety of taste to keep you on the nutritional straight and narrow.

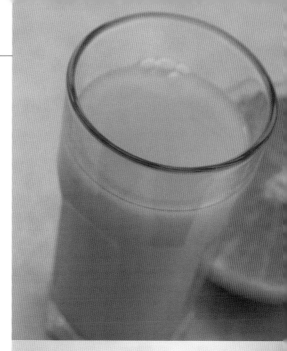

Sensible food stocks

No matter what your personal body type, you should always keep a stock of certain foods in your fridge, freezer and larder, and a fairly comprehensive list of necessities follows below. Note that you will need to adjust the quantities and suggested amounts to suit your rate of personal consumption and bodily requirements.

Remember, however, that having a well-stocked kitchen does not give you permission to consume the lot in one go!

The sensible fridge

You've started on your way to obtaining a new, and more healthy, look, and I will now give you some examples of what a sensible, weight-training person should keep in the refrigerator. Remember that you can mix and match items of food that are suitable for your particular body type.

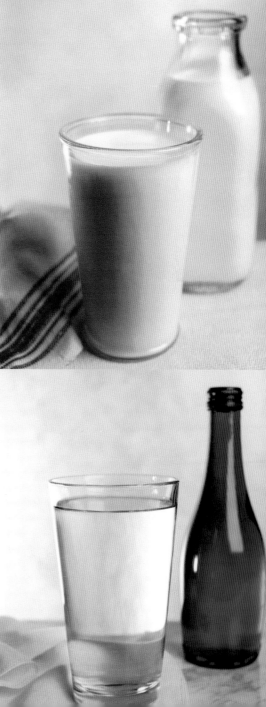

- Drinks like full-fat or semi-skimmed milk, orange juice and high-energy sports drinks are all excellent for boosting your energy. Shop-bought vegetable juices (which usually consist of around five different vegetables) are great, too, but try experimenting by making one yourself, tailored to your own tastes.

- A large bottle of mineral water that can be drunk chilled after exercising is also recommended. Dietary life doesn't have to be boring, and you could also store beers, wines and spirits in your fridge. Remember that the important factor is not what you consume, but how much.

- Meat and seafood are valuable sources of protein, and here are some suggestions for a well-stocked fridge: lean bacon (not streaky), boneless turkey or chicken breasts, extra-lean mince, the occasional beefsteak (but be warned that this tends to sit in the stomach for some time while the body absorbs it), prawns and shellfish.

- Dairy products are other good protein sources, but you'll need to take their fat content into account. Reduced-fat cheeses like Edam are a good choice, as are cottage cheese, yoghurts (always buy the low-fat varieties) and reduced-fat cream substitutes, all of which offer ways of incorporating taste and variety into your diet.

- Eggs: the perfect nutritional packages!

The sensible freezer

The sensible freezer should contain the following items:

- sufficient meat for four meals;

- unbreaded fish fillets;

- chicken breasts;

- extra-lean sausages and extra-lean steaks;

- whole-wheat bread;

- whole-wheat, low-fat waffles;

- ready-prepared meals for one or two dinners, such as low-fat burgers, vegi-burgers or any other low-fat, preprepared dish;

- vegetables of any type, perhaps broccoli, spinach, cabbage or Brussels sprouts;

- berries (such as blueberries, strawberries, raspberries, blackberries and perhaps some more exotic types), which are useful for making fruit shakes and as toppings for ice cream and other desserts;

- low-fat vanilla ice cream or yoghurt.

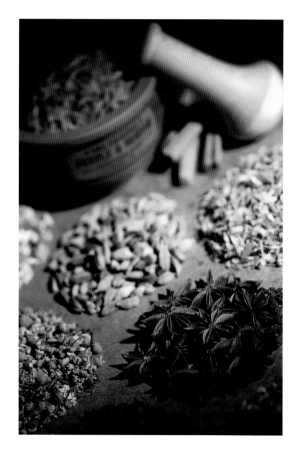

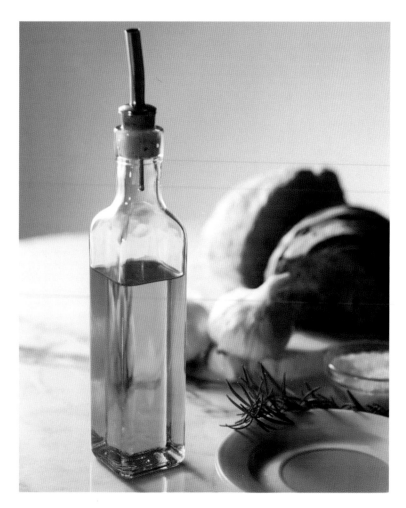

The sensible larder

The sensible larder should contain the following items.

Staples

Stock up on these ever-useful ingredients:

- oils: vegetable and olive oil;

- vinegars: malt and red-wine vinegar;

- herbs: perhaps parsley, rosemary, basil, thyme, garlic and Mediterranean seasoning;

- spices: maybe chilli, cinnamon, cumin and blends of spices like curry powder;

- flour;

- sugar;

- salt;

- pepper;

- soy sauce;

- stock cubes: beef, chicken, vegetable or all three;

- pasta; spaghetti, linguine or any other sort;

- rice.

Drinks

Depending on your personal preferences, stock up with tea, coffee or cocoa. Teas like English breakfast or Earl Grey possess antioxidant properties.

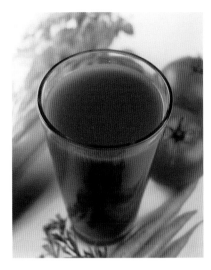

If you fancy a change from tea or coffee, not only is juice a wonderful alternative, but a freshly made juice will give your body all of the goodness it needs in one glass. The exact ingredients of your preferred juice are completely up to you, but don't be afraid to experiment with your blender and to try out some different fruit combinations. Strawberries, bananas, pears, peaches, apples and more exotic fruits, such as kiwis, paw-paws, papayas and star fruits, can all be combined with semi-skimmed milk or natural yoghurt to make a tasty, and very healthy, smoothie for breakfast.

Ready-prepared foods and tinned products

You'll always find the following items useful:

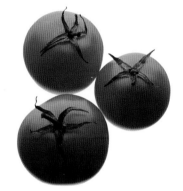

- pasta sauce (low fat);
- whole tomatoes, tomato sauce and tomato purée (low-fat);
- tinned or packet soups;
- starch- or carbohydrate-providers, such as rice, black beans, macaroni, couscous, ravioli, baked beans or, indeed, any tinned product that incorporates a sauce (always keep a stock of baked beans, chilli beans, black beans and chickpeas, all of which are valuable nutritional sources, especially if you are a vegetarian);
- tinned fruit, such as pears, strawberries, pineapples, peaches and prunes (preferably in their own juice rather than in syrup).

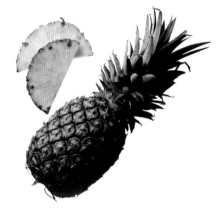

Ready-to-eat items

Make sure that your kitchen cupboards contain the following ready-to-eat items:

- a varied stock of cereals, such as branflakes, cornflakes and any wheat- or rice-based cereal (cereal bars provide a good breakfast alternative);
- raisins and nuts, such as cashew nuts and unsalted peanuts;
- crackers (whichever type you prefer);
- healthy, low-fat crisps or chips, such as tortilla chips.

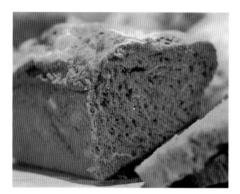

Bread

Bread is a valuable source of carbohydrates. Although wholemeal bread is preferable, the occasional slice of white bread won't hurt you.

Fruit

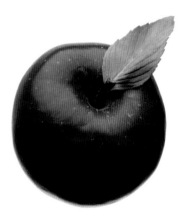

Fruit is nature's healer, providing you with all of the vitamins your body needs when following a healthy, well-balanced dietary regime and weight-training programme. I particularly recommend apples, pears, peaches, plums, melons and grapes. Berries, such as strawberries and blueberries, are very wholesome, too, but the most perfect of all is the humble banana – definitely the ideal snack before, and during, training.

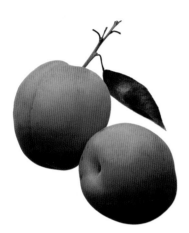

Every week you should consume at least fifteen (yes, fifteen!) servings of fruit, but if you find it hard to consume this amount, remember that your blender is your friend and that juicing fruits will give you their goodness, but not their bulk.

Vegetables

It is important to stock up with enough vegetables to provide a salad and a cooked vegetable for each of the week's home-cooked meals. I recommend buying the following:

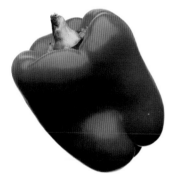

- one head of a leafy lettuce like romaine, one head of an iceberg lettuce or ready-prepared bags of lettuce;
- cucumber;
- tomatoes;
- celery;
- carrots;
- green, red or yellow peppers;
- onions;
- potatoes;

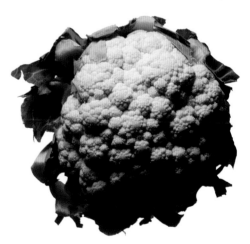

- cooking vegetables, such as broccoli, cabbage, Chinese cabbage, green beans, and aubergines;
- fresh root ginger.

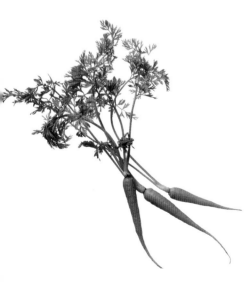

Vegetarians

Those who describe themselves as vegetarians fall into one of the following main groupings:

- semi-vegetarians, who usually exclude red meat from their diets, but often eat poultry, fish and seafood for their protein;

- ovo-lacto vegetarians, who exclude all flesh from their diets, but will eat eggs and dairy products;

- lacto-vegetarians, who exclude eggs and flesh from their diets, but will consume dairy products;

- vegans, or strict vegetarians, who eat no products derived from animals at all;

- macrobiotic vegetarians, who eat vegetables, beans, sea vegetables and whole cereal grains.

Vegetarian weight-lifters need to consume more protein than non-vegetarians. This can be derived from such plant proteins as nuts, grains and tofu, while the wide range of vegetarian products on the market today can easily sustain a vegetarian's protein requirements.

Vitamin and mineral supplements

I am not a fan of vitamin and mineral supplements. A wholesome, well-balanced diet should provide your body with all of the vitamins and minerals it needs. Although some people swear that these supplements have a beneficial effect, in my opinion it is likely to be psychological rather than physical. In short, I believe that there's no point in being a 'vitamin junkie' because popping commercially available pills has only one effect: that of emptying your wallet!

Supplements

Contrary to popular belief, relying on powdered milk-shake supplements to deliver your dietary requirements throughout the course of a busy working day is not totally forbidden. It should, however, be pointed out that not only do these liquid supplements tend to be very expensive, but many are bulked out with fibre, which has no nutritional value whatsoever, but removes any desire to eat for a considerable time after the milk shake has been consumed.

If you embark on this route, it is still important to remember the 'little and often' rule: regularly taking a lot of small sips of your supplement is far better than consuming it all in one go. This method of drinking a supplement would particularly suit a 'hard-gainer', or ectomorphic type, especially if the supplement is combined with healthy, small, well-balanced meals (see page 21).

Relying solely on supplements to meet your daily nutritional needs is not recommended, however (you'd also find it an extremely dull and expensive exercise).

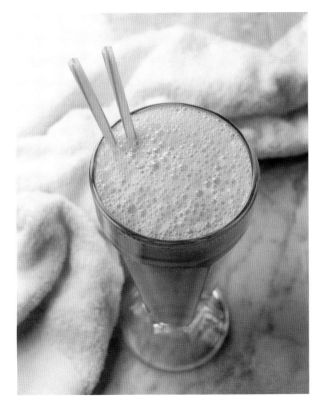

Creitine

Creitine is natural substance that has become a popular weight-training supplement used by many athletes. If you follow their example, you should not, in my opinion, expect phenomenal muscle-building results. In fact, I can tell you from personal experience that the ingestion of this supplement is far more likely to lay down reserves of fat rather than quality muscle.

Taking a supplement may also actually suppress your body's natural ability to produce this substance, making its value dubious at best. If you are taking creitine and then stop, however, your body will soon adapt and start producing its own creitine again.

Trying to obtain creitine through diet is very impractical when you consider that a healthy, balanced eating plan provides you with only 1g of creitine a day.

Hormones

Hormones are naturally occurring chemicals produced by the body, of which it generally manufactures enough. Using hormonal supplements as a short cut to attaining the body beautiful is therefore totally unnecessary.

Two of the most common hormones used for muscle-building are androstenedione (commonly known as 'andro') and DHEA, both of which pose considerable health risks. Androstenedione causes liver and heart problems, breast enlargement, personality and psychological disorders and acne. DHEA has similar side effects and also can cause irritability, prostate cancer and hair loss and disrupt the heart's rhythm. I therefore have only one piece of advice regarding taking hormones: forget it!

Blow-outs

A sensible diet should contain a balance of many varied foodstuffs, and the secret of staying on track is undoubtedly planning ahead. Don't forget that no food is bad (with the exception of saturated fats). It's the amount consumed that makes a particular item of food detrimental to the workings of your physical system.

If you are reading this book, your willpower is probably strengthening, and you'll probably be able to resist the tempting, mouth-watering treats that will soften your physique. I can, however, assure you that there will be days when you really will feel like having that chocolate bar, tub of ice-cream or beer. If so, don't worry about it. Have it! Remember that it's not what you consume, but how much, or how often, you consume it, so that the occasional blow-out won't do you any harm. Having a treat once in a while won't hurt you, and could even do your state of mind no end of good, so go ahead and enjoy yourself!

The exercises

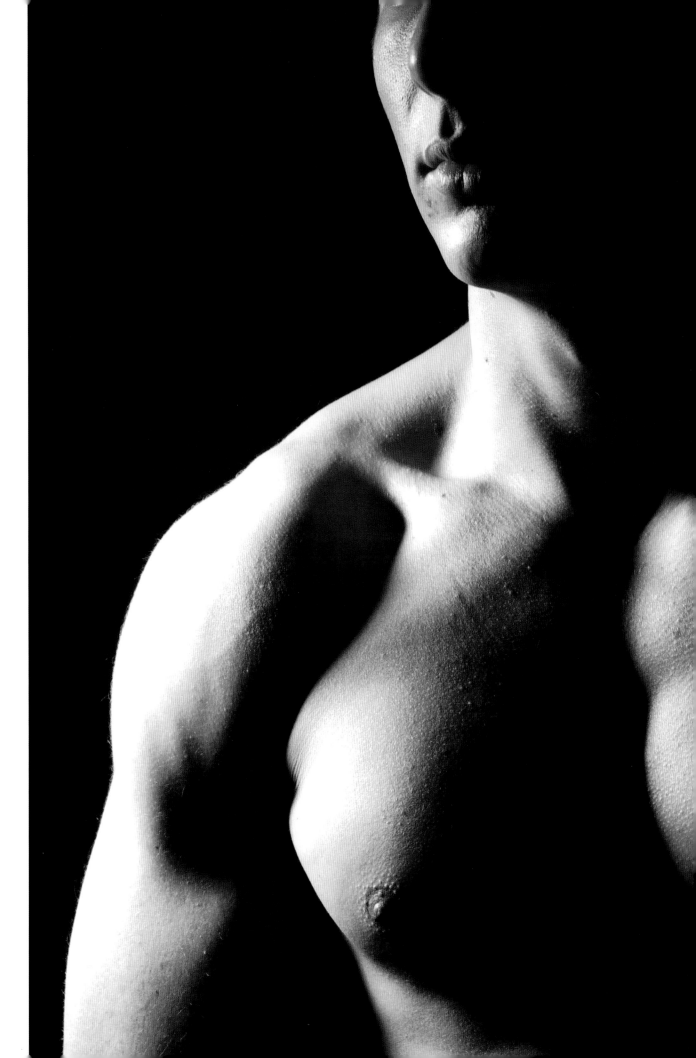

The exercises in this book provide a basic guide to fitness. They can be used in any order and, in fact, it is a good idea to mix and match your exercises and to experiment freely to find out which you prefer. Remember, too, that it is important to vary your routine sometimes to prevent boredom, the great enemy of dedication. Whichever exercises you chose to do, it is also vital that you exercise your whole body, not just part of it. You do not have to do your exercises in one session either, but could split your exercise routine, possibly exercising the top half of your body one day and the bottom half the next.

Another tip: even though the exercise routines in this book are set out in anatomical order, from top to toe, from shoulders to calves, this is only for ease of reference. You can start at any point, other than with the arm exercises. I advise leaving exercising the arms to last because your arms are used in most exercise moves and you do not want muscle fatigue to set in too early in your routine. This advice applies especially for the dumbbell and barbell curls, for which both heavy and light equipment are used.

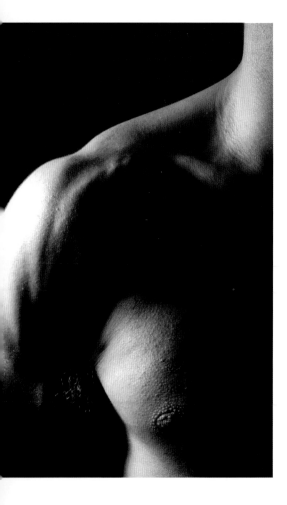

Exercising the shoulders

You'll find powerful shoulders an asset whenever you use your arms or upper body in an exercise. Every upper-body exercise involves the shoulders, so by building these muscle groups you will be able to lift heavier weights when developing your chest and back.

Exercising these muscle groups is a prerequisite to achieving a well-defined form, too. Massive shoulders define a man's physique, giving a 'V'-shaped appearance. (You only have to look at a manual worker to see shoulders that are well developed and defined.) Shoulders that are large and well proportioned give the illusion that the waist is narrow: if you possess enormous shoulders, your waist will seem to shrink in proportion, even if it measures 91.5cm (36in).

Many people who have just started weight-training are overly enthusiastic and can easily injure the muscles that form the shoulders, however. This is why it is particularly important to have your training partner close at hand when performing certain shoulder exercises to avoid failure. (This is also a good rule to follow when performing all of the exercises included in this book.)

When exercising your shoulders, *never* arch your back! Although arching your back will give you extra power and leverage, the risk of injuring your lower back becomes intolerably high and must definitely be avoided. Remember that a lower-back injury is very painful, and that if you incur one you will be unable to exercise any muscle group at all for a considerable amount of time.

The muscles of the shoulders

The shoulder muscles are called the deltoids, a name that means 'triangular in shape'. These muscle groups allow you to lift, rotate and extend your arms. The deltoids are further subdivided into the front, back and side deltoids.

Like those in the abdominal region, the groups that comprise the shoulder muscles should be exercised separately. Always remember that these muscles are particularly prone to injury during workouts and that you should therefore take extra care when exercising them.

Exercise 1: front-deltoid raises

This is a great exercise for muscle-building because it works the upper-arm muscles, trapezius and pectorals, along with the shoulders.

Always keep the weight that you use on your dumbbells low to start with. As well as never overloading your dumbbells, take this exercise gradually and build up your strength over a period of time.

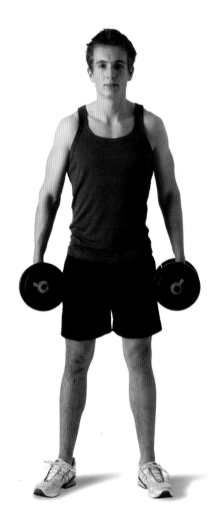

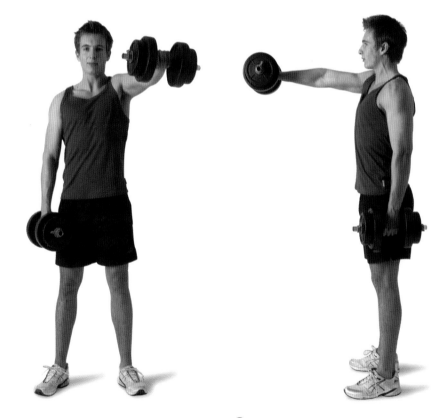

A Stand up straight, with feet a shoulder-width apart and knees slightly bent. Hold a dumbbell in each hand and allow your arms to hang at your sides, elbows slightly bent. Your palms should be facing your upper thighs. Lean forward *very slightly* at the waist, keeping your elbows back, your chest pushed out and your lower back straight.

B Slowly raise your left arm in front of you until it is at shoulder height. The palm of the hand that you are working should be facing downwards. *Never* rock your hips or swing your arms to gain momentum. Hold the position for a few seconds and then slowly return to your starting position.

C Finish the set and switch arms.

Exercise 2: bent-over lateral raise

This exercise is designed to enhance the back deltoid muscles.

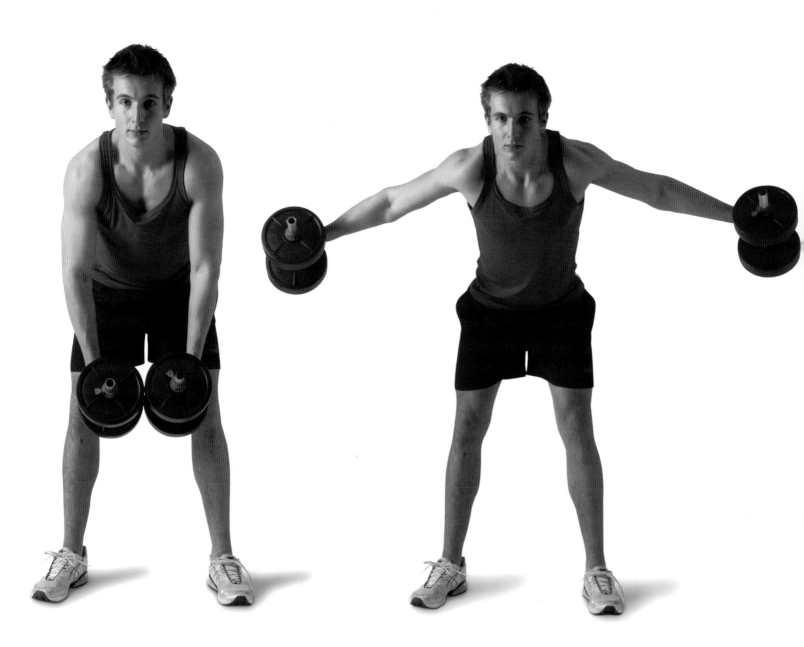

A Holding a dumbbell in each hand, bend over at the waist, with your arms in front of you and your elbows slightly bent. Your palms should be facing each other. Your feet should be a little more than a shoulder-width apart. *Always* keep your back straight and roughly parallel to the floor.

B Slowly raise the dumbbells in unison out towards your sides, as if you were flapping your arms. Raise your arms until they are parallel to the floor, remembering *always* to keep your back straight. Hold the position for a few seconds and then slowly return to the starting position.

Exercise 3: behind-the-neck press with barbell

This all-purpose exercise targets the back deltoids, pectorals, upper-back triceps and ribcage muscles. It is equally effective when performed at the front of the neck, which, in my opinion, is the much safer option and is dealt with in Exercise 4: overhead press with barbell. If you like, you could alternate both variations.

In accordance with the rule of gradually building up your resistance to the weight, it would be a good idea to use lighter weights than usual for this exercise.

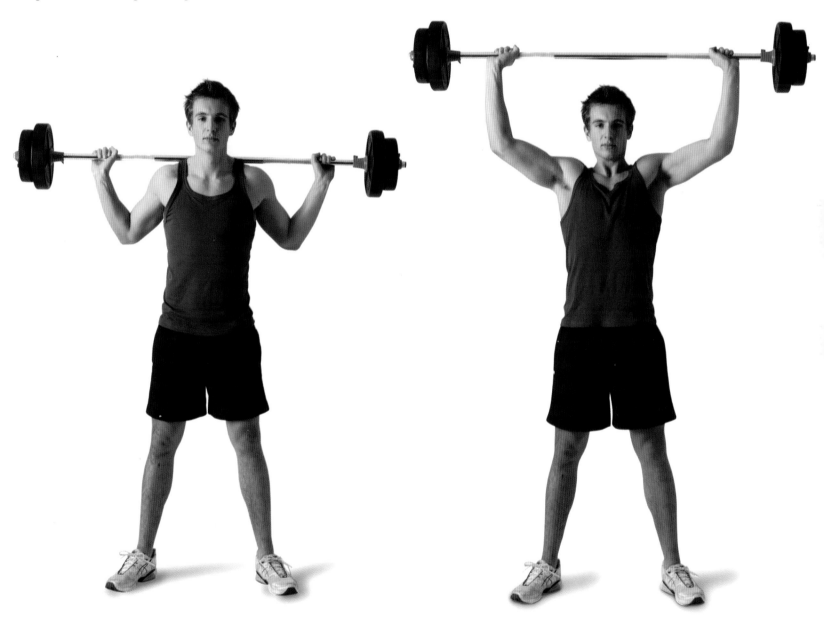

A Stand with your back straight and your feet a shoulder-width apart. Bend your knees slightly. Position a barbell behind your neck, across the top of your shoulders. Your hands should be slightly more than a shoulder-width apart, with the palms facing forwards. Keep your elbows pointed downwards and your chest extended. *Never* arch your back!

B Keeping your elbows pointing outwards, slowly raise the barbell straight upwards. Pull your head forward slightly to give the barbell space in which to move. Hold the position for a second and then slowly lower the barbell to the starting position.

Exercise 4: overhead press with barbell

This exercise targets the front and side deltoids. It can be alternated with
Exercise 3: behind-the-neck press with barbell.

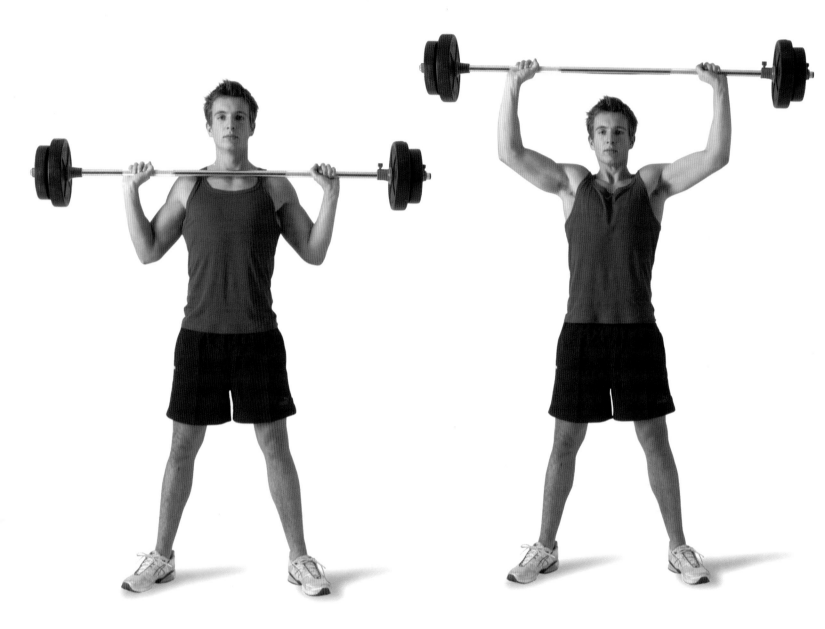

A   Stand with your back straight, your feet a shoulder-width apart
    and your knees slightly bent. Hold the barbell overhand, with
    your hands a shoulder-width, or slightly further, apart. Bend your
    elbows and raise the barbell to shoulder level. Keep your elbows
    pointing downwards and your chest extended.

B   Slowly lift the barbell straight over your head. Hold the position
    for a second and then slowly lower the barbell to chest level.

Exercise 5: shrugs

Apart from developing the shoulders, this exercise strengthens your rhomboids, which lie between your spine and shoulder blades.

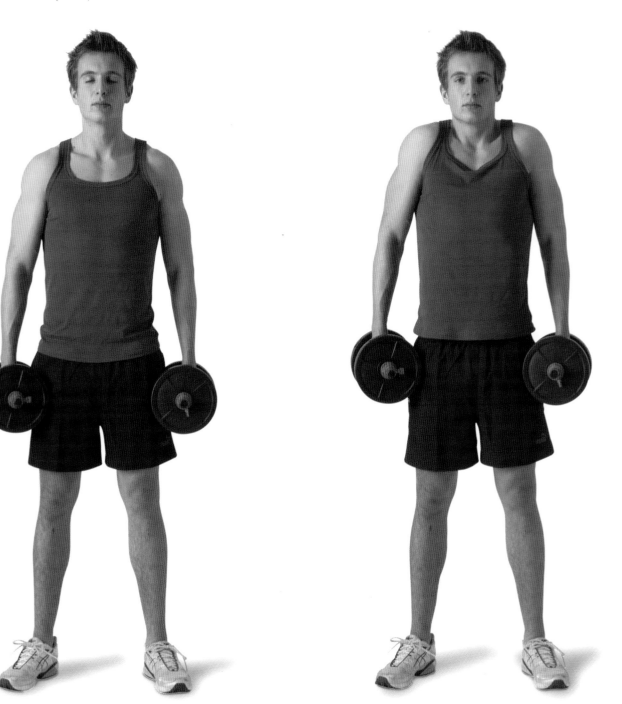

A   Stand up straight, with your feet a shoulder-width apart and your knees slightly bent. Holding a dumbbell in each hand, allow your arms to hang alongside your body. Your palms should be facing inwards, towards your body. Make sure that your shoulders are held back and *never* tense them – in other words, relax!

B   Slowly shrug your shoulders as high as they will go, keeping your head still and your chin tucked in slightly. Hold the position for a second and then slowly return to the starting position.

Exercise 6: dumbbell military press

This exercise works your front and side deltoids, as well as your trapezius and triceps. Because your arms must work alone, remember to use less weight than you would for an overhead press.

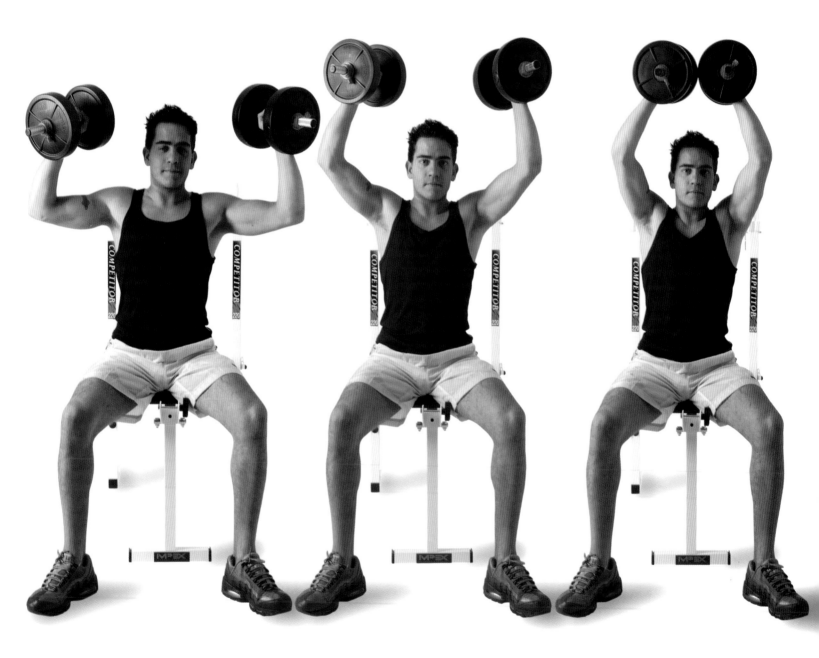

A   Sit on the end of your bench, holding your back completely straight. Take a suitably weighted dumbbell in each hand. Your palms should be at shoulder height and facing inwards.

B   Slowly raise both dumbbells over your head until they are almost touching.

C   Extend your arms fully and *never* allow your elbows to lock. Pause for a second and then slowly lower the dumbbells to the starting position.

Exercise 7: upright rowing

As well as developing your shoulders, this exercise is excellent for strengthening your biceps and forearms.

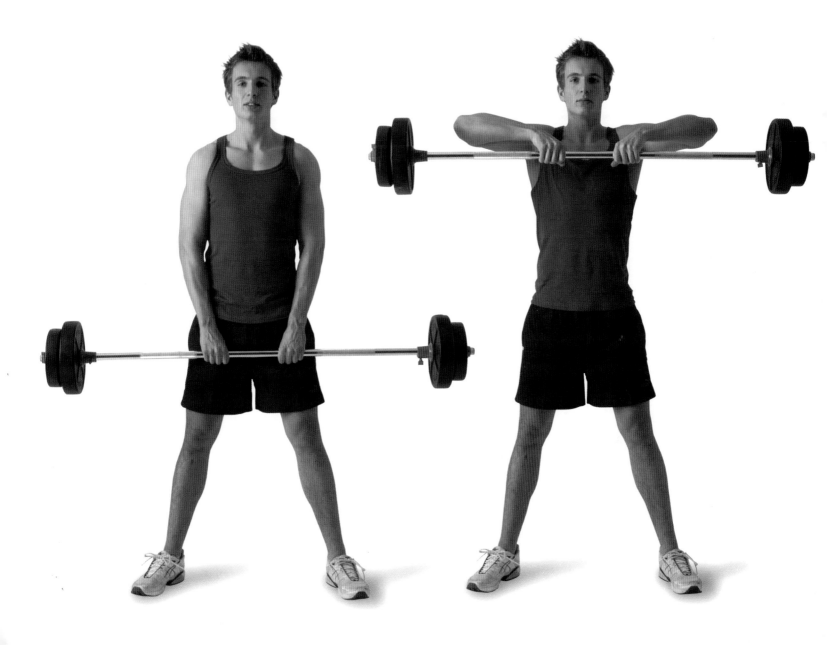

A Stand upright, holding a barbell in both hands using a narrow grip, with your palms facing downwards. Your arms should be fully extended in front of you, with the barbell level with your upper thighs. Relax your shoulders slightly, but remember always to keep your back straight.

B Slowly pull the barbell straight upwards and tuck it under your chin. Your elbows should be pointing upwards and outwards. Hold the position briefly and then slowly lower the barbell to the starting position.

Exercise 8: dumbbell raise

In addition to working your side deltoids and trapezius, this exercise builds the rhomboids, pectorals and biceps.

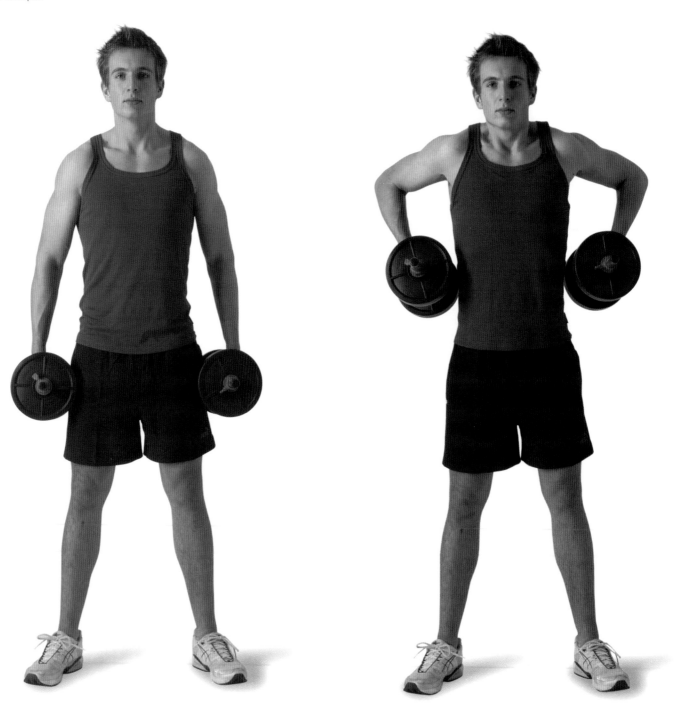

A   Stand with your back held straight and your legs a shoulder-width apart, with your knees slightly bent. Holding a dumbbell of a suitable weight in each hand, with your palms facing towards your body, let your arms hang down by your sides.

B   Slowly raise the dumbbells as far as you can towards your armpits. Without jerking at the top of the lift, keep your elbows pointing outwards and the dumbbells close to your body. Hold the position for a few seconds and then slowly lower your arms to the starting position.

Exercise 9: side-deltoid raise
This exercise targets your side deltoids.

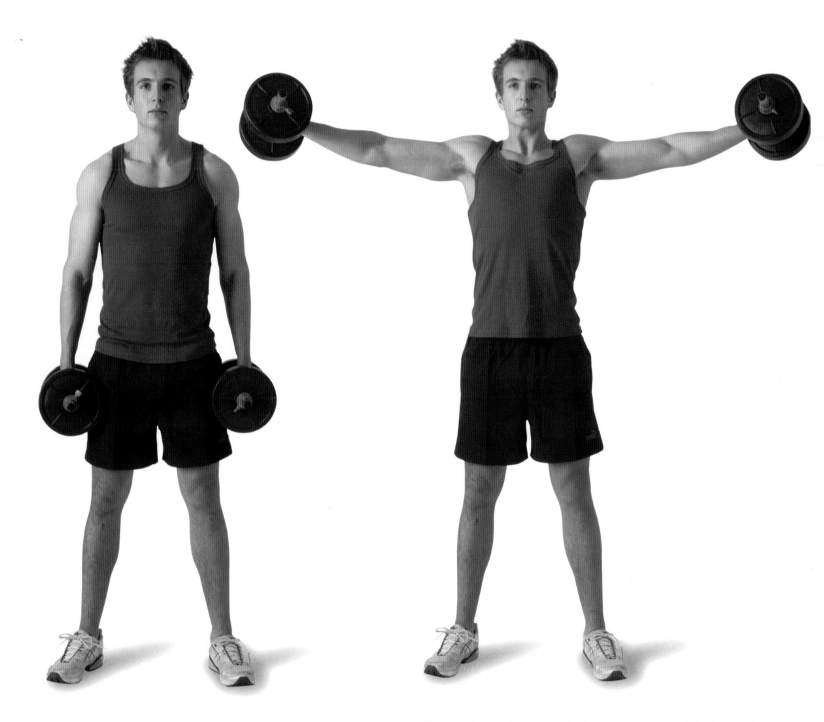

A Hold a dumbbell in each hand, with your arms by your sides, your palms facing towards your body and your elbows slightly bent. Stand upright, with your feet a shoulder-width apart. Keep your shoulders back, your chest extended and your lower back straight, but with a slight lean.

B Slowly raise both dumbbells in unison in a straight line until they are at shoulder level. Ensure that your elbows remain slightly bent, at the same time keeping your arms in the same plane as your torso. Hold the position for a second and then slowly lower your arms to the starting position.

Exercise 10: front-deltoid raises with weight

In addition to working key shoulder muscles, this exercise builds your trapezius, chest and inner upper-arm muscles.

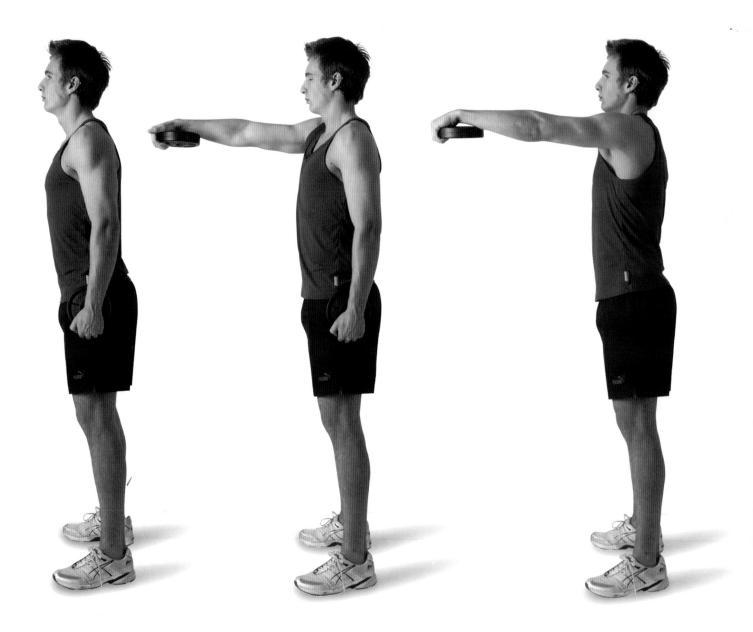

A   Stand up straight, with your feet a shoulder-width apart and your knees slightly bent. Hold a disc of a suitable weight in each hand and allow your arms to hang by your sides, with your elbows slightly bent and your palms facing your upper thighs. Lean forward slightly at the waist, keeping your elbows back, your chest extended and your lower back straight.

B   Slowly raise your right arm in front of you until it is at shoulder height. The palm of your hand should now be facing downwards. *Do not* swing your hips or rock your arms to gain momentum. Hold the position for a second and then slowly return to the starting position.

C   Repeat the exercise once using your left arm and then alternate arms.

Exercise 11: pull-up (no weight)

This exercise is a great workout for the rhomboids, the muscles that lie between your spine and your shoulder blades, as well as for the latissimus dorsi in your back.

You'll need a specialised piece of equipment called a chin bar, a relatively inexpensive item that can be temporarily, yet securely, fixed within a doorway of your home.

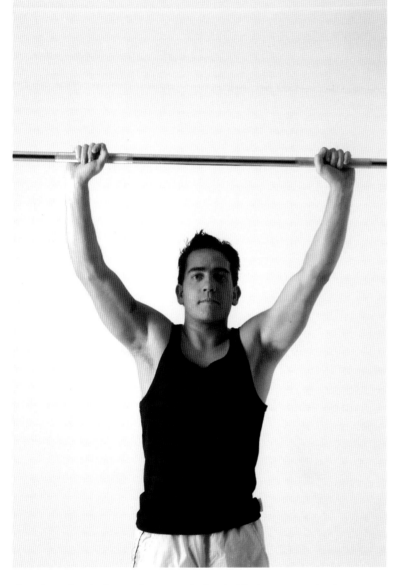

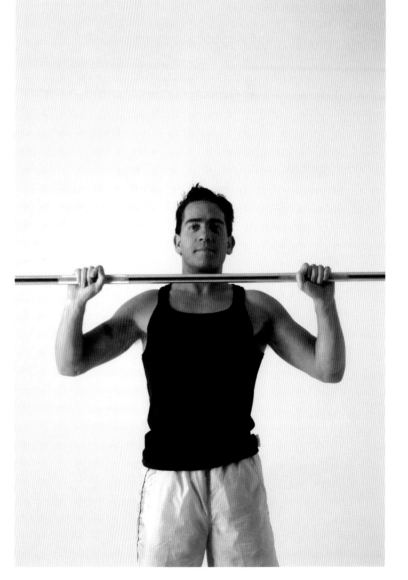

A   Standing in front of a securely fixed chin bar, grasp the bar overhand, with your hands about 45 to 50cm (18 to 20in) apart. Remember that your feet should not touch the ground at any time during this exercise.

B   Using a slow, steady motion, pull yourself up until your chin is higher than the bar. Hold the position for a second, then slowly lower yourself to the starting position. Exhale on the way up and inhale on the way down. *Do not* swing your body to gain momentum.

Exercise 12: dumbbell raise

In addition to working your side deltoids and trapezius, this exercise builds the rhomboids, pectorals and biceps.

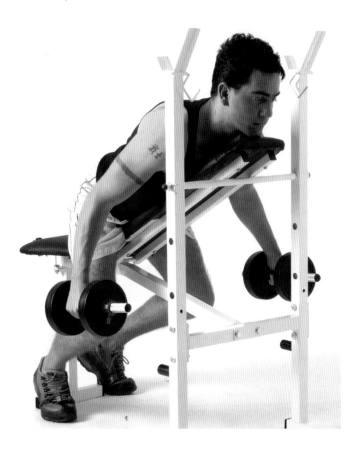

A   Stand facing an incline bench, with your chest against the incline. Your legs should be a shoulder-width apart, with your feet on the floor and your chin just above the top of the bench. Holding a dumbbell in each hand, keep your elbows slightly bent and your palms facing each other as you let your arms dangle below the level of the bench.

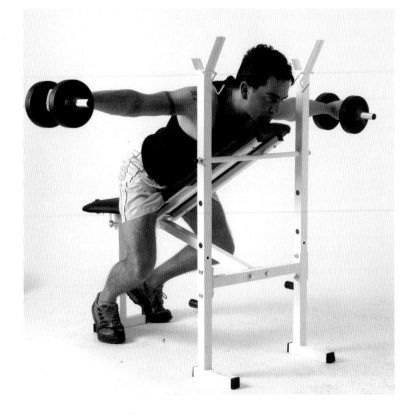

B   Keeping your elbows relaxed, slowly raise your arms to the sides until they are at approximately shoulder height. Hold the position for a second and then slowly return to the starting position.

Exercising the arms

Nothing grabs the attention more than large, well-formed arms, and most men would like to possess arms like Hercules' or Atlas'. Taken together with the other top muscle groups, such as the pectorals, abdominal and shoulder muscles, the upper arms give a defined look overall and a well-balanced appearance.

Big arms are an essential asset to any serious weight-trainer, which is why male weight-trainers usually concentrate on the muscles of the upper arms more than any others. These arm muscles are fortunately one of the easiest groups to develop successfully.

The arms are worked especially hard in upper-body exercises. A good training tip is to work your arms last, particularly after an upper-body workout, because they may otherwise have become exhausted by your previous efforts and could fail you just when you need them the most. The last thing that you want is to lose arm strength and power when performing really heavy repetitions for your chest and back.

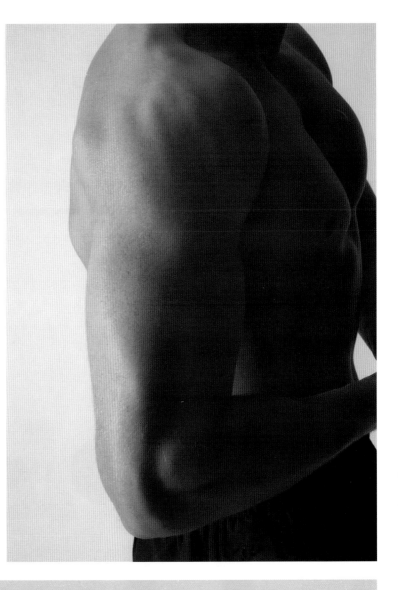

The muscles of the arms

The muscles of both the upper and lower arms are part of the 'flexor' muscle group that enables you to bend your arms and bring your hands to your shoulders. You may be interested in the following facts about each of the muscle groups in the arms.

The biceps (a word that means 'two heads') are actually two muscles. The bicep brachii is located on the top of the upper arm and provides the 'head' of the muscle, while the larger brachialis, together with the triceps, supports the under arm.

The lower arm, or forearm, consists of three main muscle groups, the brachiora dialis, the flexors and the extensors that permit you to bend your wrists and extend your fingers. Powerful forearms help to lift weights and give a strong grip. Most men's forearms develop very easily indeed. Because every upper-body exercise inevitably involves a gripping action, the forearms and wrists benefit almost as a side effect of other routines. Unless you participate in sports that require a firm grip, such as rock-climbing, golf, tennis or even arm-wrestling, you therefore need not develop your forearm muscles separately.

Exercise 1: hammer curl

This exercise works the elbow flexor muscles or biceps on the front of your arms.

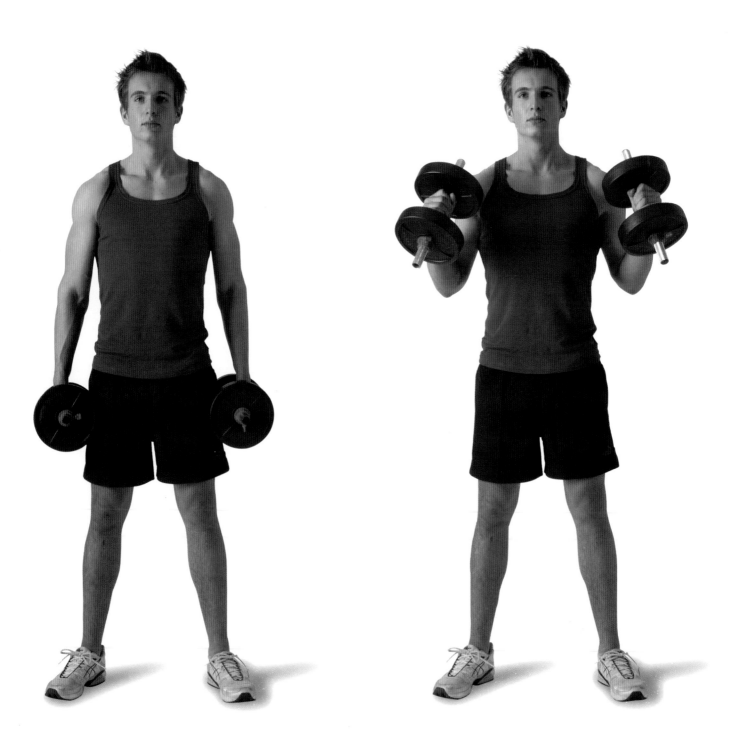

A Stand up straight, with your feet a shoulder-width apart and your knees slightly bent. Holding a dumbbell in each hand, with your palms facing inwards, extend your arms fully.

B Slowly curl the dumbbells until the ends touch your shoulders. *Never* rotate your wrists while curling, but *do* keep your upper arms and elbows stationary. Hold the position for a second and then lower the dumbbells slowly, using a controlled motion, to the starting position.

Exercise 2: concentrated curl

This exercise works the other elbow flexors in the arm.

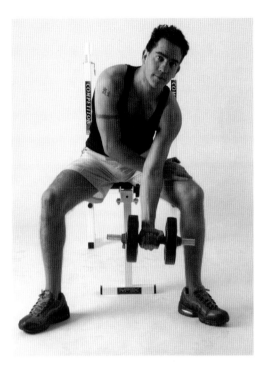
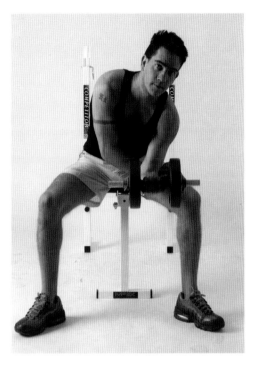
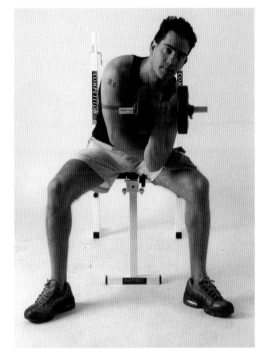

A   Sit on either a solid, sturdy chair or on the end of a weights bench, with your feet slightly more than a shoulder-width apart. Hold a dumbbell in your left hand, with your arm fully extended and your palm facing upwards. Rest your left elbow on your left inner thigh and your right hand on your left upper thigh. Bend forward slightly, *always* keeping your back straight.

B   Slowly curl the dumbbell upwards, towards your shoulder, keeping your upper arm vertical in relation to the floor.

C   Hold the position for a second and then slowly lower the dumbbell, using a controlled motion, to the starting position.

Always finish the set before switching arms and repeating the exercise.

Exercise 3: barbell curl

This movement strengthens the elbow flexors.

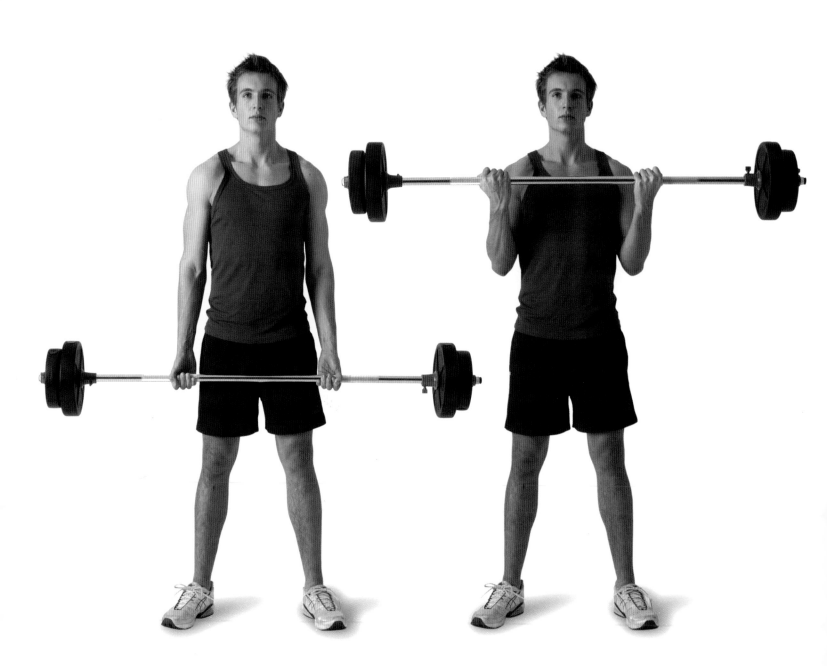

A   Stand up straight, with your knees slightly bent. With your hands a shoulder-width apart and your palms facing upwards, hold a barbell underhand. Your arms should be extended and the barbell should be level with your thighs.

B   Keeping your elbows close to your body, use your biceps to curl the barbell slowly towards your chin. Keep your wrists straight throughout the curl and *never* sway your back or rock your body to gain momentum. Hold the position for a second and then slowly return to the starting position, using a smooth, controlled motion.

Exercise 4: reverse-grip barbell curl

This is an excellent exercise for the flexor muscles at the front of the arms.

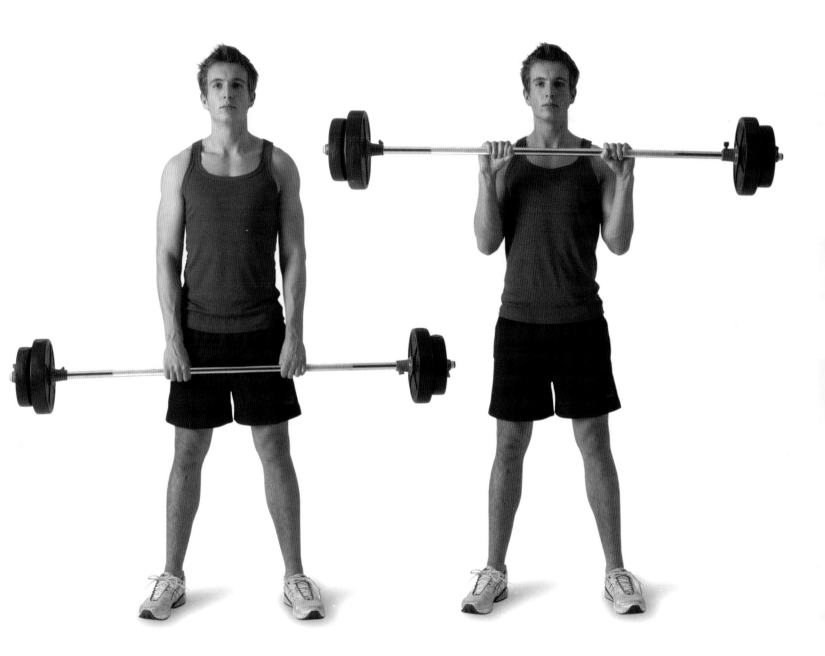

A Stand up straight, with your feet a shoulder-width apart and your knees slightly bent. Hold the barbell in an overhand grip, with your hands spaced a shoulder-width apart. Your arms should be fully extended, with the barbell resting against your upper thighs. Keep your elbows tucked in at all times.

B Slowly curl the barbell towards your chin. Hold the position for a second at the end of the lift, then slowly lower the barbell to the starting position, using a smooth, controlled action.

Exercise 5: alternating dumbbell curl

This exercise also gives the elbow flexors a good workout.

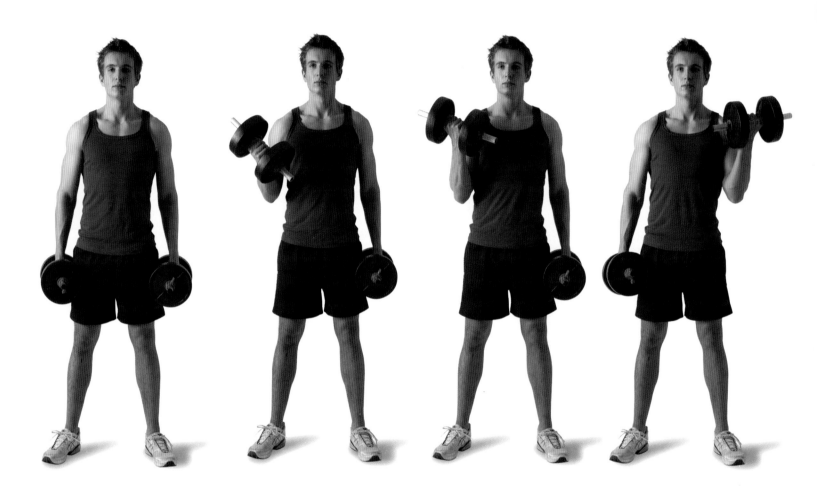

A Stand up straight, with your feet a shoulder-width apart and your knees slightly bent. With your arms by your sides and your palms facing inwards, hold a dumbbell in each hand.

B Slowly curl the right dumbbell upwards, towards your collarbone. As you perform the curl, rotate your arm so that your palm now faces upwards.

C Hold the position for a second at the top of the lift and then slowly lower the dumbbell, using a controlled motion, to the starting position.

D Repeat the exercise using your left arm.

Exercise 6: inclined dumbbell curl

This exercise gives the biceps a good workout.

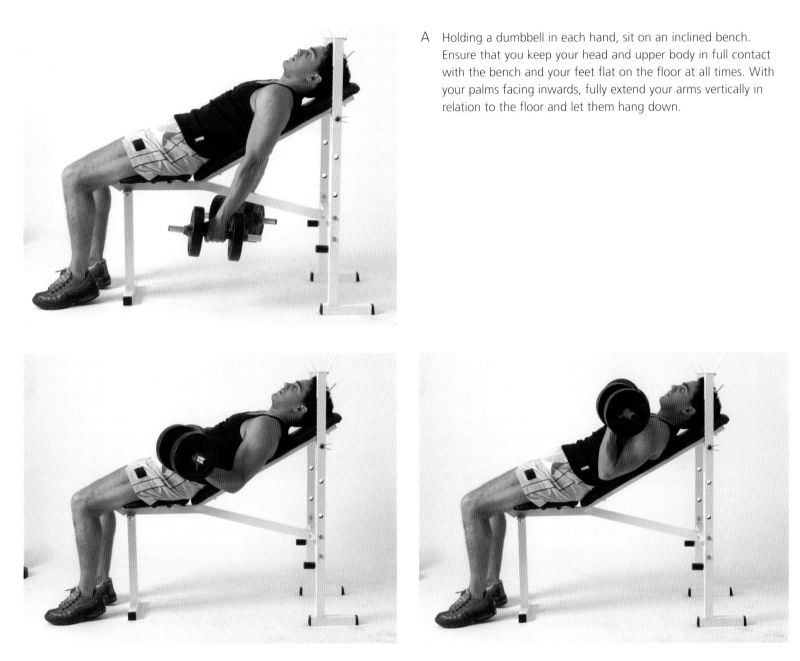

A Holding a dumbbell in each hand, sit on an inclined bench. Ensure that you keep your head and upper body in full contact with the bench and your feet flat on the floor at all times. With your palms facing inwards, fully extend your arms vertically in relation to the floor and let them hang down.

B Slowly curl both dumbbells upwards, toward your shoulders, keeping your upper arms stationary and your elbows pointing downwards.

C Your palms should rotate upwards during the lift until they face your shoulders. Hold the position for a second and then slowly lower both arms to the starting point, using a smooth, controlled action.

Exercise 7: seated overhead triceps extensions

This exercise works the extensor muscles at the back of the arms. For safety's sake, if you are using plates that can be removed from your dumbbell, ensure that the collars are *always* tight.

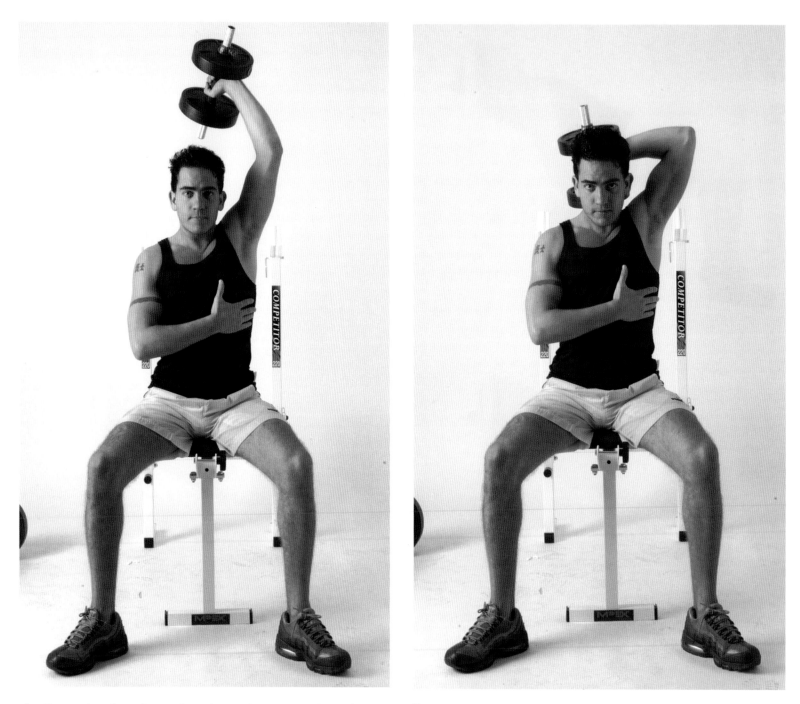

A   Sit on a bench, with your feet planted firmly on the floor. Using one arm, and with your palm facing upwards, hold a dumbbell over your head. Keep your back straight, although your lower back should be inclined forwards slightly.

B   Keeping your upper body in position and your upper arm close to your head, slowly lower the dumbbell behind your head, using a controlled, semi-circular motion, until your forearm is as close to your biceps as possible. You may lean forward slightly to help you to balance the weight, but *never* sway or arch your back. Your elbow should be facing forwards. Hold the position for a second, then slowly return to the starting position, using a smooth, controlled motion.

Exercise 8: lying triceps extension

This movement works the elbow extensors. It is important always to use a little weight at first and then to build it up slowly. It is also crucial always to ensure that the collars are tight on dumbbells with removable plates.

A Lie on your back on a weights bench, with your head extending slightly over the end of the bench and your feet flat on the floor. With both of your thumbs around the bar, hold a dumbbell so that the full weight is resting on your palms. Extend your arms at an approximately 180° angle, but don't lock them. The weight should be over your head. Keep the dumbbell bar vertical.

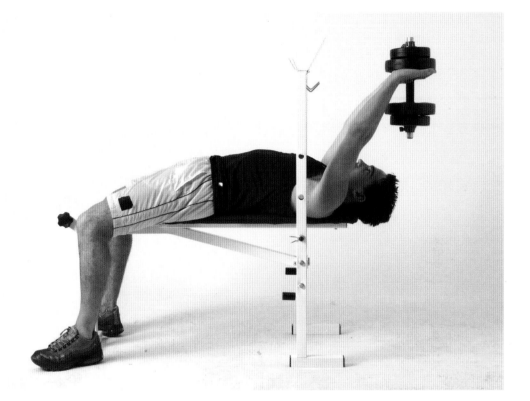

B Slowly bend your elbows as you lower the weight until it is behind your head. Hold the position for a second and then slowly return to the starting position, using a smooth, controlled motion.

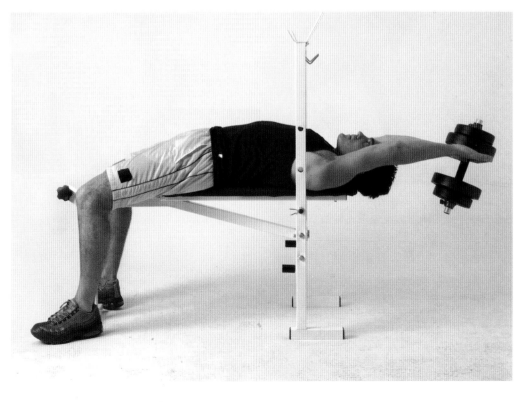

Exercise 9: dumbbell kick-back

This exercise works the elbow extensors.

A Holding a dumbbell in your left hand, support yourself on an exercise bench with your right knee and right hand. Keep your left foot firmly on the floor. Your back should be straight and parallel with the floor. Your left arm should be bent at an angle of 90°.

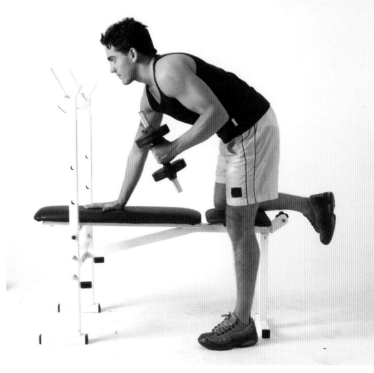

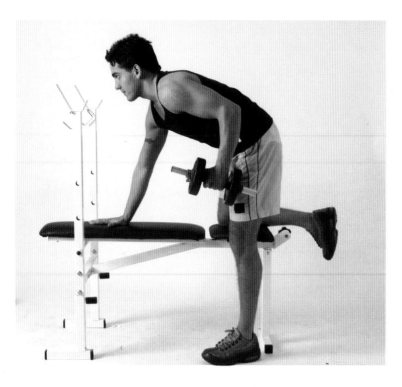

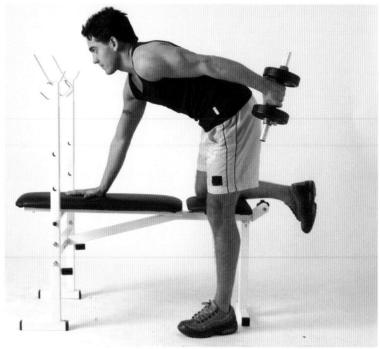

B Slowly straighten your left arm and extend the dumbbell behind your body, keeping your upper arm parallel with the floor.

C As you are doing this, you should feel your left arm's triceps muscle contract fully. Then slowly bend your left arm again, bringing the dumbbell back to the starting position.

Finish the set and then switch to your right arm.

Exercising the chest

The chest is considered to be one of the most attractive features in both sexes. And a well-balanced chest will both aid you in pushing and provide a powerful look: a barrel-chested man can give the impression of being totally impervious to harm, even something of a superhero.

A well-developed chest therefore evokes a very powerful image indeed, and in order to achieve this much-desired result, you must alternate at least eight different chest exercises, utilising as many angles as possible to work many different muscle fibres. Building strong triceps and deltoids will provide an overall sculpted look, thereby adding to the impressiveness and definition of your chest.

The following section gives you all of the information you need to build up your chest in the old-fashioned, and, in my opinion, best-possible way, that is, by using free weights.

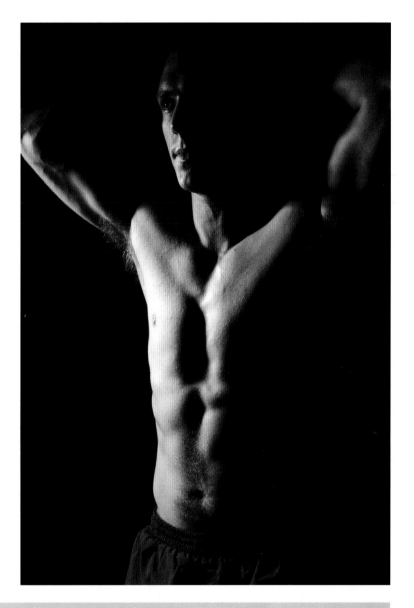

The muscles of the chest

The muscles of the chest consist of the pectoral major and the pectoral minor. The pectoral major is the larger muscle, joining your shoulder, collarbone and breastbone. The pectoral minor is located beneath its larger counterpart.

You may also hear talk about upper and lower pecs and clavicular upper, and sternal lower, chest fibres, but this really just blinds you with science. The important thing is to concentrate on the major and minor pectorals.

In my opinion, the best way of bulking up your chest muscles is to perform the bench press (Exercise 1), the incline dumbbell bench press (Exercise 2) and the decline bench press (Exercise 3), remembering to include as many angles in your chest-exercise routine as possible. It is important to realise that variation and angle are the key ingredients in gaining an impressive chest. When you start to feel the 'twitch' of your chest fibres, you will know that you are on the right track.

Exercise 1: bench press

This classic exercise (for which it is important to have a training partner), also works your deltoids and triceps.

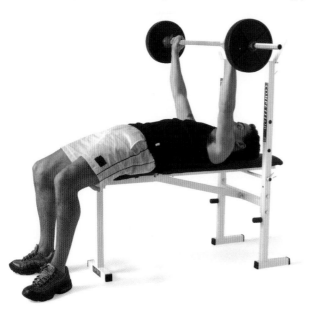
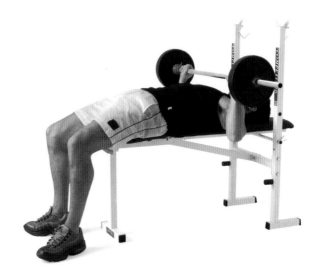

A   Lie on a weight-training bench, with a barbell above your chest. Grasp the barbell with your hands, which should be about a shoulder-width, or slightly further, apart. Your palms should be facing your legs, and your feet should be resting on the floor. Keep your back straight and pressed against the bench.

B   Slowly lower the barbell to your nipple line. Your elbows should be pointing downwards, while the rest of your body remains in position. Don't arch your back or bounce the barbell off your chest. Hold the position for a second, then slowly raise the barbell to the starting position.

Exercise 2: incline dumbbell bench press

This exercise builds your triceps. It is best performed with a training partner to hand.

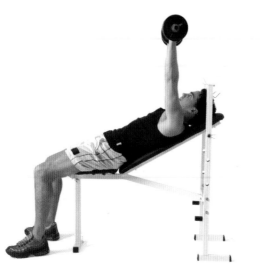
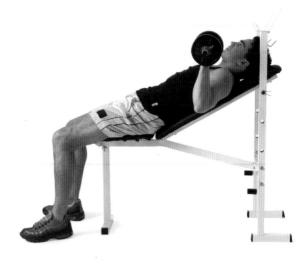

A   Lie on a 45° incline bench, with your arms fully extended and perpendicular to the ground. Hold a dumbbell overhand in each hand, with your palms facing your feet, your arms a shoulder-width apart, your back pressed against the bench and your feet flat on the floor.

B   Slowly lower the dumbbells to your shoulders, keeping your elbows pointing outwards. Pause for a second, then slowly extend your arms again in a controlled motion. Try not to arch your back or bounce the dumbbells off your chest at the bottom of the lift.

Exercise 3: decline bench press

This is similar to a regular weight-training press, but stresses the lower portion of the pecs.

Caution

This is a difficult, and potentially dangerous, move. Use weights that are lighter than your usual weights, and be sure to have a training partner with you. In fact, to avoid injury, use especially light weights until you have mastered the movements.

A   Lie on a decline bench, with your head under the barbell rack and your knees bent, or hanging over the far end of the bench. With your arms a shoulder-width apart, hold the barbell using an overhand grip, with your palms facing your feet. Lift the bar off the rack and hold it straight above your chest.

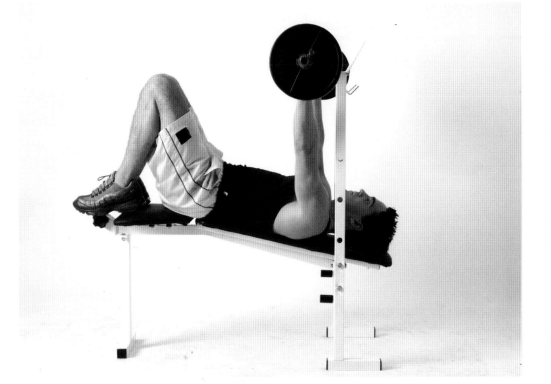

B   Slowly bend your elbows, lowering the barbell to just below your nipples, always keeping your elbows pointing outwards. Hold the position for a second, then slowly press the barbell back up in a controlled motion, extending it to arm's length.

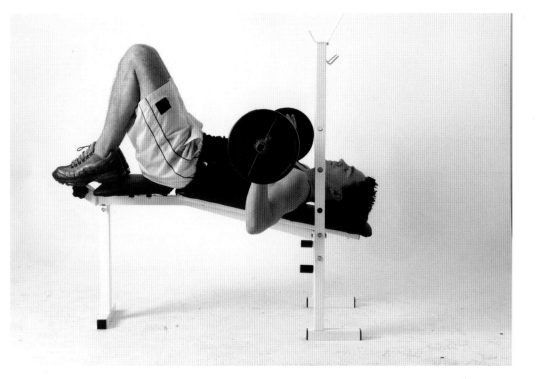

Exercise 4: barbell overhead pull

This exercise, for which you should use light weights, works the latissimus dorsi in your back, as well as your rhomboids
and shoulder-blade muscles.

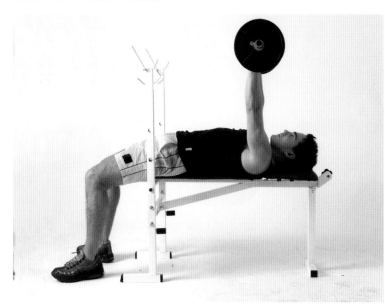

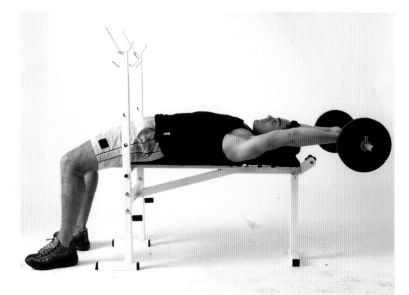

A   Lie flat on a bench, with your feet placed on the floor on either side. With your palms facing your feet, lift the barbell above your chest until your arms are perpendicular to the floor, keeping your elbows unlocked and slightly bent.

B   Slowly lower the barbell behind your head in a semi-circular motion until your upper arms are parallel to the bench or lower. Don't let your elbows form an angle of less than 90°. Hold the position for a second, then slowly pull the barbell back over your head to the starting position.

Exercise 5: dumbbell fly

This move also works your shoulder adductors from your chest to your inner arms, as well as the flexors across the front
of your shoulders.

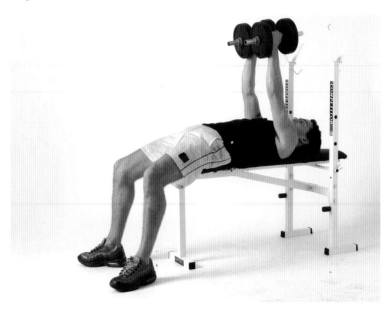

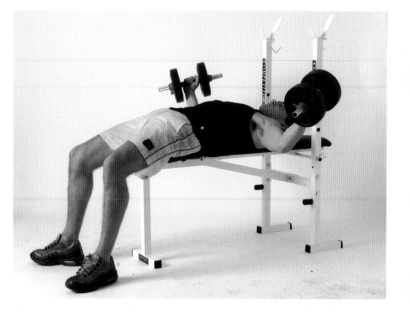

A   Lie on your back on a bench, with your legs parted and your feet placed firmly on the floor. With your palms facing each other, hold two dumbbells above your chest so that they are nearly touching each other. Your back should be straight and pressed firmly against the bench. Don't lock your elbows.

B   Using a semi-circular motion, slowly lower the dumbbells outwards, away from each other, until they reach chest level. Keep your wrists locked, your elbows bent at an angle of roughly 90° and your back straight. Hold the position for a second, then slowly raise the dumbbells to the starting position.

Exercise 6: dumbbell bench press

This exercise works your triceps slightly more than a barbell weight-training bench does. Like the barbell version (see Exercise 1, page 66), a training partner should be present for this exercise.

A   Lie flat on a weight bench, with a dumbbell in each hand and your arms fully extended, perpendicular to the floor. The ends of the dumbbells should almost touch each other. Your feet should be flat on the floor and your palms should be facing your feet. Keep your head and body in full contact with the bench.

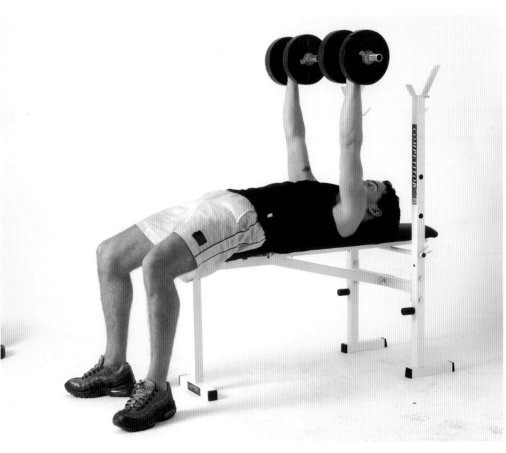

B   Slowly bend your elbows and lower your arms straight downwards, until the dumbbells are just above the sides of your chest. Pause for a second, then slowly raise your arms back up again. Keep the dumbbells under control and don't let them bounce or arch your back.

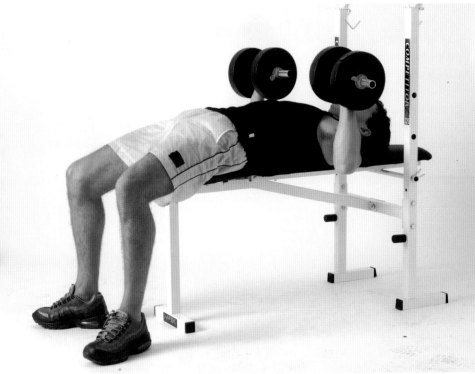

Exercise 7: bent-arm pull-over

This move also strengthens the latissimus dorsi muscles of your back, as well as your triceps. Use lighter weights than normal until you get used to it. If the dumbbell weight plates are removable, make sure that the collars are tight before beginning.

A   Lie across a bench, with your head extending just beyond the end. Keep your torso straight and your feet flat on the floor. Hold a dumbbell by the end, with your palms facing upwards and your thumbs around the bar. Your arms should be extended above your chest, with your elbows slightly bent.

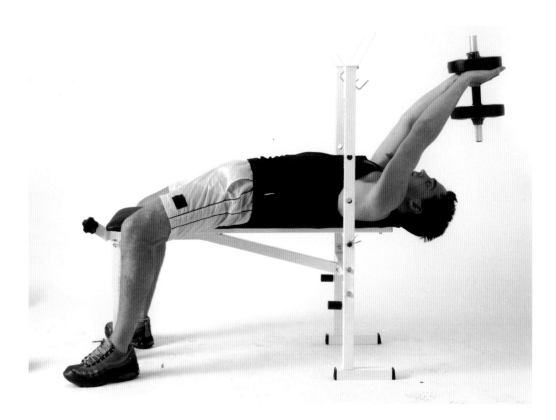

B   Slowly lower the dumbbell backwards over your head until your upper arms are parallel with the floor. Don't arch your back. Pause for a second, then slowly raise the dumbbell back to the starting position.

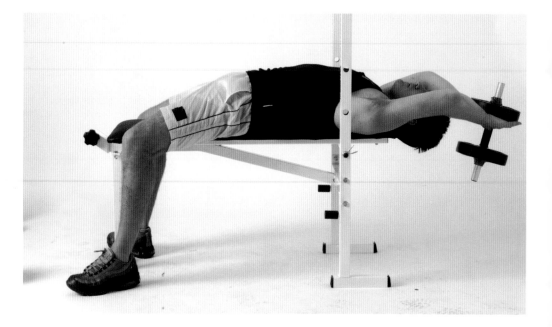

Exercise 8: push-up

This classic exercise also strengthens your shoulders, arms, wrists and upper back.

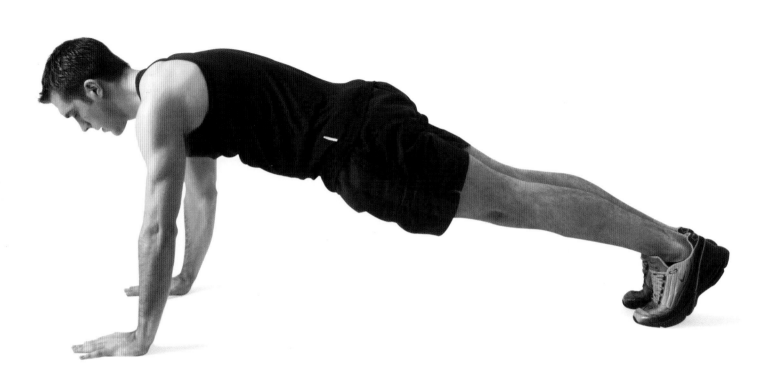

A   Lie face down on the floor, balancing your weight on the balls of your feet and the palms of your hands. With your hands a shoulder-width apart, extend your arms fully, but don't lock your elbows. Keep your legs together and fully extended and your fingers pointing forwards. Make sure that your legs, back and neck are in a straight line and keep your eyes on the floor.

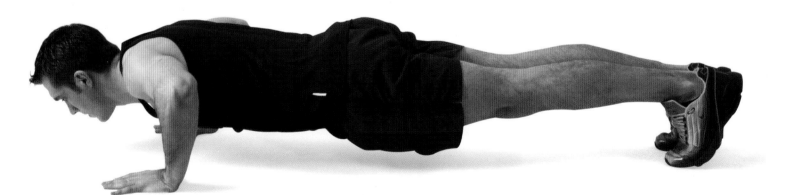

B   Slowly bend your arms, keeping your body straight and lowering yourself until your chest almost touches the floor. Hold the position for a second, then slowly return to the starting position.

Exercise 9: decline push-up

This is a more difficult variation on the standard push-up.

A Assume the standard push-up position (see the previous page), with your legs together and arms and legs extended, but instead of putting your feet on the ground, rest them on a weight bench. Keep your elbows slightly bent and your fingers pointing forwards. Keep your eyes on the floor and your legs, back and neck in a straight line.

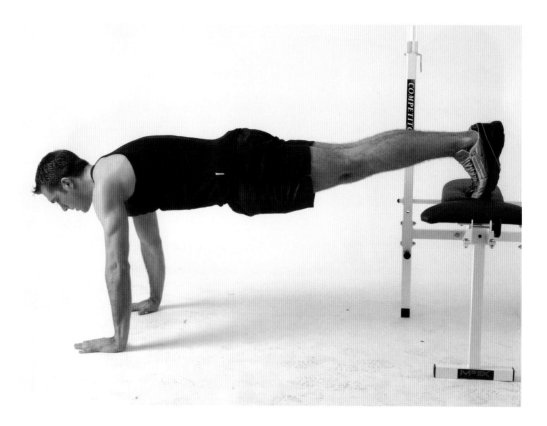

B Keeping your body straight, bend your arms, slowly lowering yourself until your chest almost touches the floor. Hold the position for a second, then slowly return to the starting position.

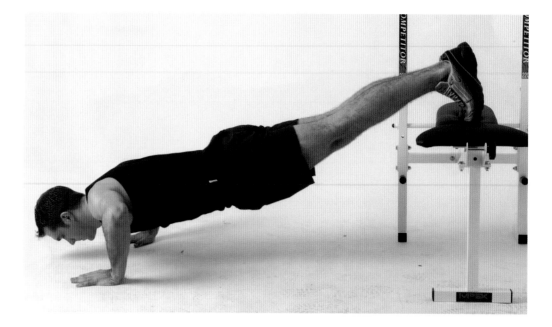

Exercise 10: one-handed push-up

This push-up variation works one side of the body at a time.

Caution

One-handed push-ups aren't for beginners. You will need very strong arms and shoulders and good balance to avoid incurring a serious injury while doing this exercise.

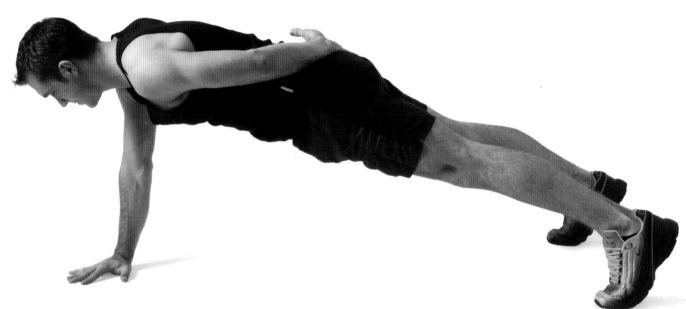

A   Place your right hand on the floor and twist your body sideways. Place your left hand behind your back. If you need to, place your left foot sideways on the floor to help you to balance. Only the toes and ball of your right foot should touch the floor. Now push yourself up with your right arm – when it's straight and supporting your body weight, you're ready to begin.

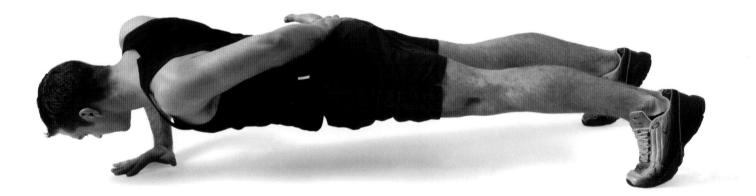

B   Slowly lower yourself until you're roughly 10 to 13cm (4 to 5in) from the floor. As you go down, you may place your free hand on your hip to help you to balance. Hold the position for a second at the bottom, then push yourself back up to the starting position.

Perform three to five repetitions, then switch arms. As your training progresses, slowly work your way up to performing more repetitions.

Exercise 11: power push-up

In this push-up variation, the emphasis is on speed (power) rather than strength.

A   Let yourself fall forwards, catching yourself before you hit the floor with your hands by assuming a push-up position. Your weight should be resting on your palms and toes. Your legs and back should be straight.

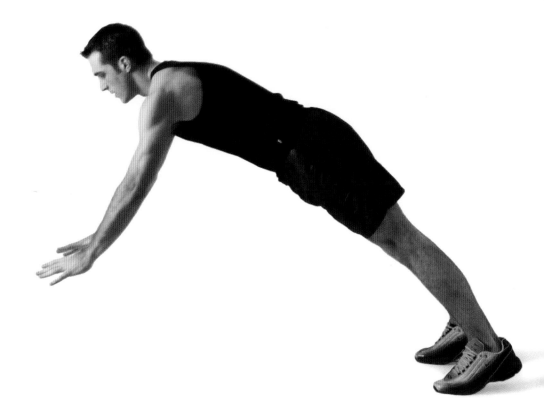

B   Immediately lower yourself and then explosively push yourself back up to the starting position.

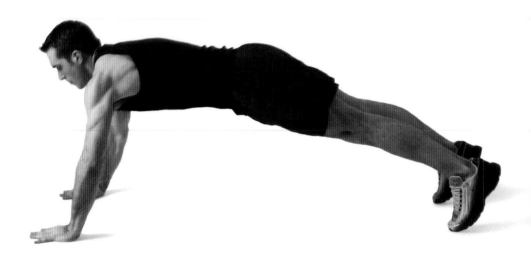

Exercising the abdomen

In my opinion, defined abdominals are among the most obvious and impressive features of an athletic man's physique. These muscle groups help to maintain a good posture and strong back. In addition to these important functions, they support the internal organs, which is why this region is sometimes called the abdominal wall.

It is vital that the abdominal muscles are kept fit. Although this is not as hard as it sounds, there is, as usual, some bad news: working these muscle groups alone will not build a perfect washboard look. The problem with this narrow approach is that even the fittest of us generally have no less than around 8cm (about 3in) of flab around the midriff, no matter how hard we try to shift it with standard exercises like sit-ups and side bends. Early morning television is full of commercials promising that this or that gadget will guarantee success in building up and defining your midriff, usually over a period of thirty days. This approach is very unlikely to earn you those admiring glances at the beach or in the baths, however, making it best to forget about faddy gizmos that promise to 'bust your gut' and instead to stick to a sensible training regime and eating plan.

It has to be emphasised that working only one part of your body will not yield the results that you crave. In order to achieve a perfect 'ripped' look, it is important to combine an aerobic exercise, such as walking, stair-climbing, jogging or cycling, with a sensible eating plan. So if you wish to attain the defined, washboard look, cakes, chocolate, pies, burgers, and all of those other mouth-watering sins that we love so much, are definitely completely out!

To develop muscles in the abdominal area, it is necessary to lose fat from the whole body through dieting so that the abdominal muscles show through clearly. It is impossible to lose fat from one area of the body alone through dieting.

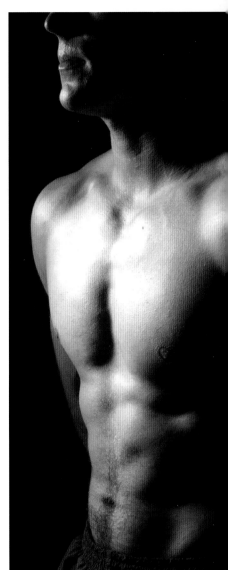

The abdominal muscle group

There are three muscle groups in the abdominal wall: the upper abs (abdominals), the lower abs and the lateral obliques, which are found on either side of this central region.

It is not advisable to exercise all of these muscles at once, or in succession, if you want to achieve the best possible results. A far better strategy is to vary the exercises for this region. In other words, if you regularly train on a Monday, Wednesday and Friday, you should alternate the exercises between these days. You could, for instance, exercise your upper abs on Monday, your lower abs on Wednesday and your lateral obliques on Friday, or in whatever order best suits your personal training regime. This will prove a far more effective method of exercising the abdominals in terms of achieving maximum results because you will give the individual muscle groups the chance to rest and recover between workouts. Also a good plan to apply to the other muscle groups in the body, this technique is generally known as 'splitting the workouts'.

Exercise 1: hip raises with ankle weights

This exercise is a good all-round workout for your abdomen because it works all of the major muscle groups in your torso. It is particularly good for working your bottom and thigh muscle groups.

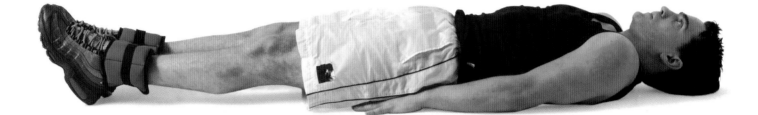

A First secure the ankle weights firmly around your ankles, and lie flat on your back on the floor.

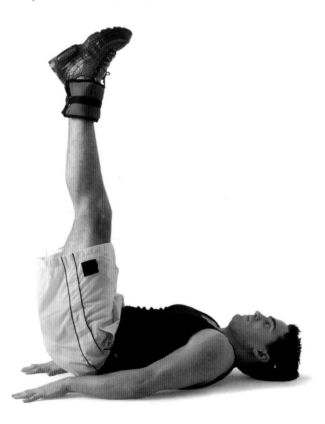

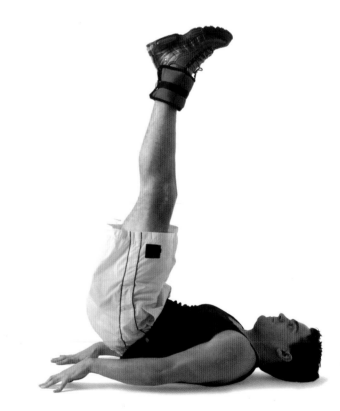

B Raise your legs in the air, keeping your toes pointed. *Do not* lock your knees! Place your arms by your sides, with your hands facing downwards.

C Tightly holding in your abdominals, shift your weight towards your shoulders. Slowly lift your hips off the floor, keeping your legs in a vertical position throughout the exercise. Hold the position for a few seconds and then slowly return to the starting position.

Exercise 2: negative sit-ups with weight plates

This move exercises both the upper and lower abdominals.

A   Sit on the floor, with your knees bent and your feet placed flat on the ground a shoulder-width apart. Now tuck your feet under a suitably secure object, such as a weights bench or sofa. (There are also special items of equipment that you could purchase for this purpose; alternatively, your training partner could hold your feet.)

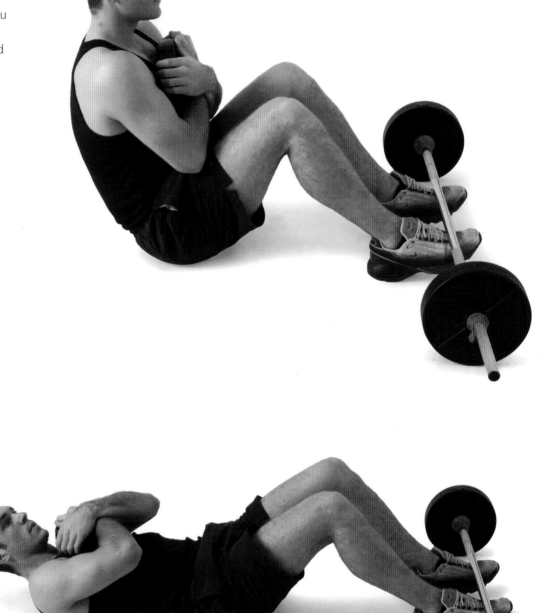

B   Place a suitable weight plate on your chest and hold it firmly in place before slowly lowering your torso almost to the floor. *Never* go all of the way down to touch the floor. Hold the position for a few seconds and then slowly raise yourself to the starting position.

Exercise 3: curl-up with weight plates

This is a great exercise for the upper and lower abdominals.

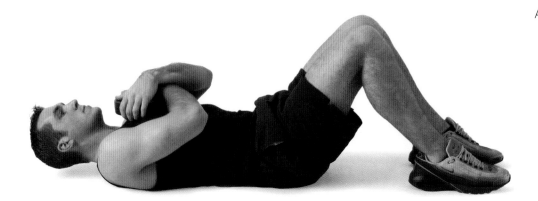

A Lie flat on your back holding a suitable weight plate on your chest, with your elbows pointed outwards. Bend your knees at an angle of approximately 45°. Place your feet a shoulder-width apart, about 15cm (6in) from your bottom. (You may find that it helps to place your feet under a suitably heavy object, such as a weights bench or sofa, for added stability; your training partner could also come in handy for this purpose.)

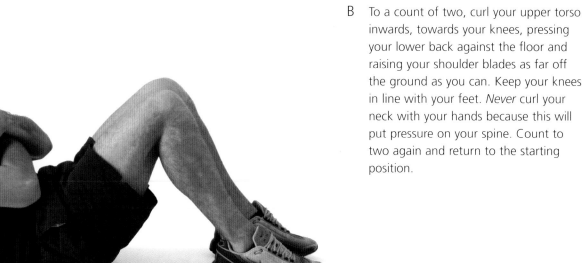

B To a count of two, curl your upper torso inwards, towards your knees, pressing your lower back against the floor and raising your shoulder blades as far off the ground as you can. Keep your knees in line with your feet. *Never* curl your neck with your hands because this will put pressure on your spine. Count to two again and return to the starting position.

Exercise 4: leg raises with ankle weights

This is a good general abdominal exercise.

A   Securely fasten an ankle weight around each ankle. Lie on your back on a weight bench, with your hips close to one end.

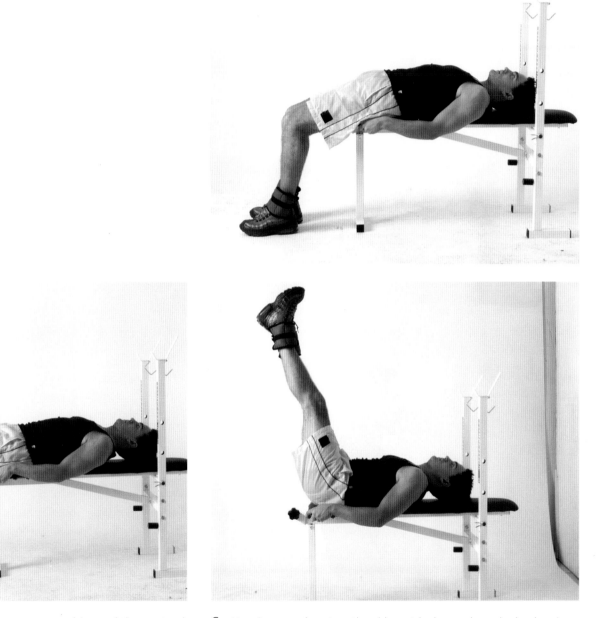

B   Grasp the corners of the bench next to your hips and then extend your legs straight outwards, pointing your toes.

C   Keeping your legs together (do not lock your knees), slowly raise them to a vertical position by pressing your back into the bench. Now slowly lower your legs, using a controlled motion, until your body is completely horizontal.

Exercise 5: rowing crunch with ankle weights

This move gives your abs a good overall workout.

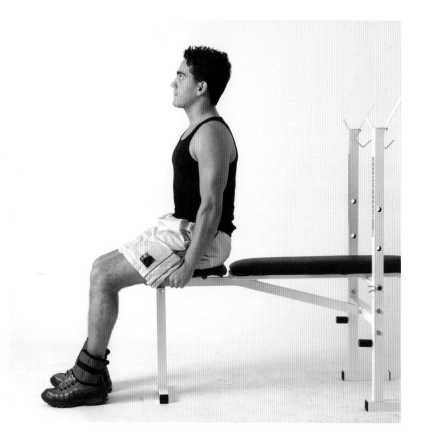

A   Securely fasten an ankle weight around each ankle. Sit on a weights bench, with your knees bent and your feet flat on the floor. Grasp the sides of the bench for support and then lean backwards, to an angle of approximately 45°. Keeping your knees slightly bent, extend your legs and raise them a few inches off the floor.

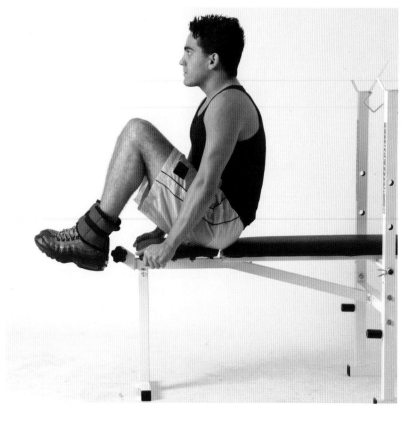

B   While bringing your body into an upright position, slowly pull your knees to your chest as far as you can without losing your balance. Hold this position for a count of two, then simultaneously return your upper body and legs to the starting position, keeping your back straight.

Exercise 6: side bends (no weight)

This exercise strengthens the muscles responsible for torso movement. Remember to keep your body facing forwards and *never* to turn your torso into a sideways twist because you may wrench your back muscles and injure yourself.

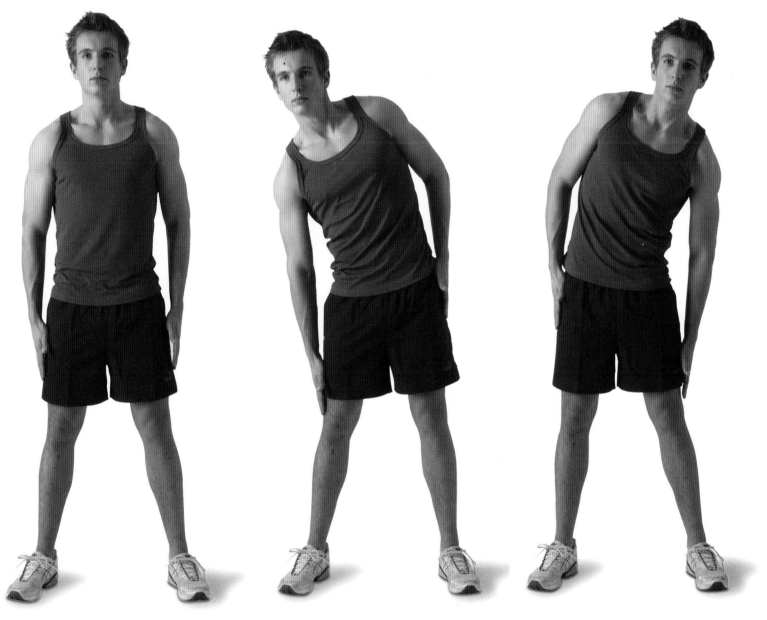

A   Stand upright, with your arms held in a natural position by your sides and your palms facing inwards. Your feet should be a shoulder-width apart.

B   Slowly bend to one side, tensing your lateral-oblique muscles until you feel them pulling. Slowly bring yourself upright again, into the starting position, and then repeat the movement.

C   Finish the set for one side of your body before repeating the exercise for the opposite side.

Exercise 6a: side bends with dumbbells

Like Exercise 6, of which it is an extension, this exercise strengthens side-to-side movement. Designed for the more advanced weight-trainer, it requires free weights to be held on either side of the body to provide more resistance while performing the set.

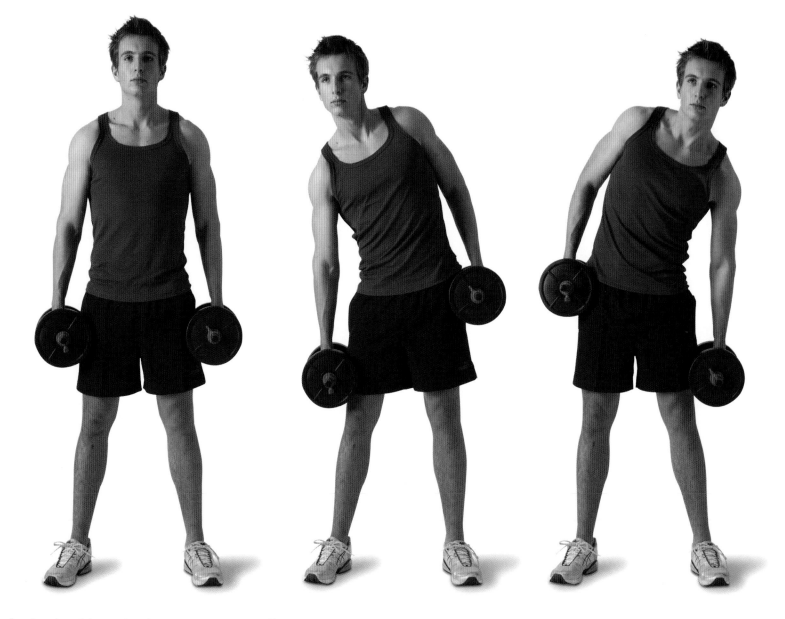

A   Stand upright, with a dumbbell in each hand and your feet a shoulder-width apart. Your arms should be resting by your sides, with your palms facing inwards.

B   Slowly bend to one side, allowing the dumbbell on that side to drop down your thigh until you feel your lateral obliques pulling. Keep your body facing forwards, in the same plane, and *do not* allow your torso to move into a twist or to rock from side to side. When you have gone as low as you can, slowly bring yourself upright again, into the starting position, keeping your abdominal muscles and lateral obliques contracted.

C   Finish the set without resting between repetitions and then repeat the set for the opposite side.

Exercise 7: seated twist

This is an exercise that will work all of the abdomen's major muscle groups. It is specifically designed for the lateral obliques, but also works the upper and lower abs. You will need a rod, or a light bar, about the length of a broomstick for this exercise.

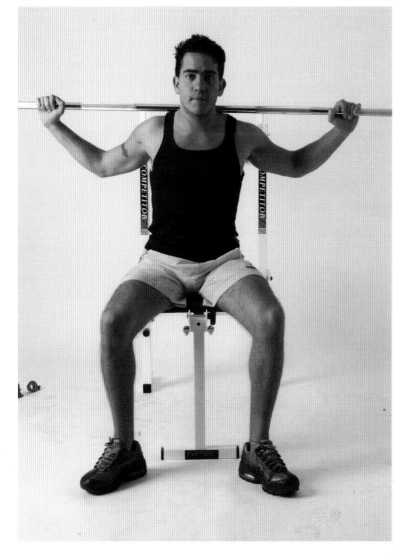

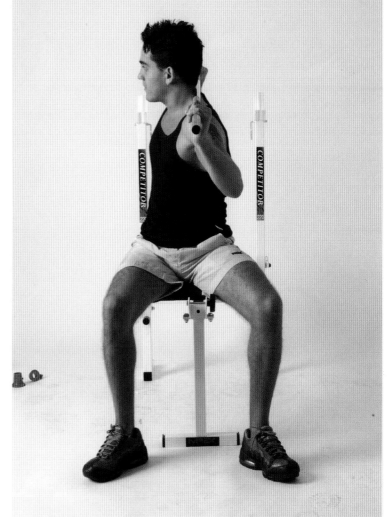

A   Sit on a weight bench and rest the bar behind your head, across your shoulders. Place your hands as close to the ends of the bar as you comfortably can, with your elbows slightly bent.

B   Use your oblique muscles to twist your torso smoothly as far to the right as you can, keeping your hips stationary. Your head should move with your torso. Repeat the same smooth movement to the left and then continue to rotate to the right and left without pausing until you have completed the set.

Exercise 8: curl-up

This exercise works the upper and lower abdominal wall.

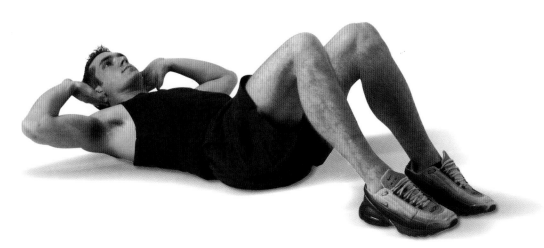

A   Lie flat on your back on the floor, with your hands cupped behind your ears and your elbows pointing outwards. Bend your knees to an angle of about 45°, with your feet positioned a shoulder-width apart and about 15cm (6in) from your bottom.

B   Curl your upper torso inwards, towards your knees, pressing your lower back against the floor and raising your shoulder blades as high as you can. Keep your knees in line with your feet and *do not* use your hands to curl or pull your neck. Move your torso all the way up in a count of two, contracting your abdominal muscles as you do so. Hold the position for a second, then slowly return to the starting position.

Finish the set without resting between repetitions.

Exercise 9: oblique trunk rotation with weight plate

Perform this exercise in one slow, continuous motion.

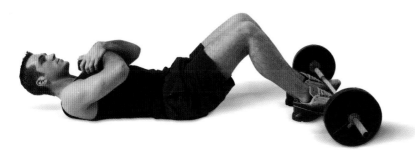

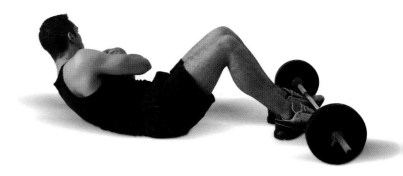

A Lie on the floor, with your knees bent and holding a weight plate against your chest. Tuck your feet under a support, such as the base of a weights machine or bench, to stabilise your lower body.

B Hold your torso at an angle of 45° to the floor.

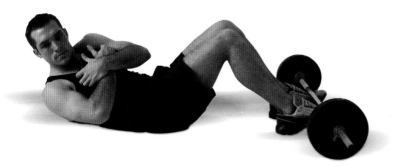

C Start by slowly moving your body to the left, keeping to the left as you lower yourself down, onto your back.

D Slowly raise your torso as you move towards your right side to complete a clockwise rotation.

Now repeat the exercise, this time moving down on your right side and around to your left.

Exercise 10: dumbbell trunk twists

This move also works your biceps and forearms.

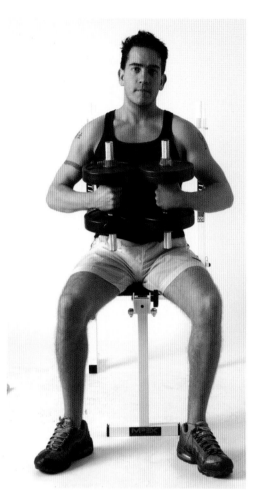 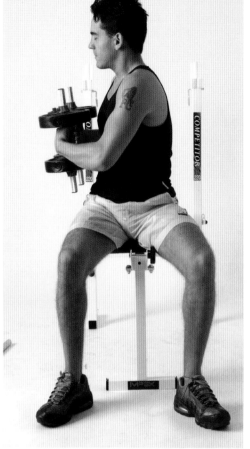 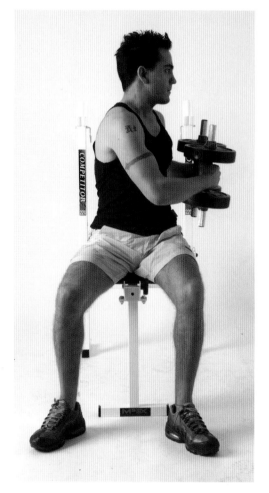

A Sit on the edge of a bench, with your feet flat on the floor. Keep your chest pushed out and your head aligned with your torso. Holding a dumbbell in each hand, with your palms facing your body, bend your arms and bring the weights close to your stomach.

B Slowly and smoothly twist your torso as far to the right as you comfortably can. When you reach the end of your range of motion, hold the position for a second, then slowly return to the starting position.

C Repeat the exercise, this time moving to your left. Continue alternating the movement to the right and left until your muscles are fatigued.

Exercise 11: hip raises (no weight)

In addition to strengthening your lower abs, this exercise works your bottom and quadriceps.

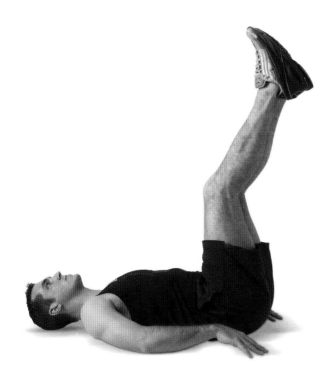

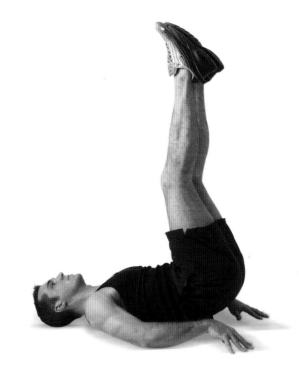

A   Lie flat on your back, with your legs in the air (don't lock your knees), your toes pointed and your hands at your sides, palms facing downwards.

B   Using your lower abs, and shifting your weight towards your shoulders, lift your hips off the floor, keeping your legs vertical throughout. Pause, and then slowly return to the starting position.

As an alternative, you can do this exercise with your legs crossed if this is more comfortable.

A   B

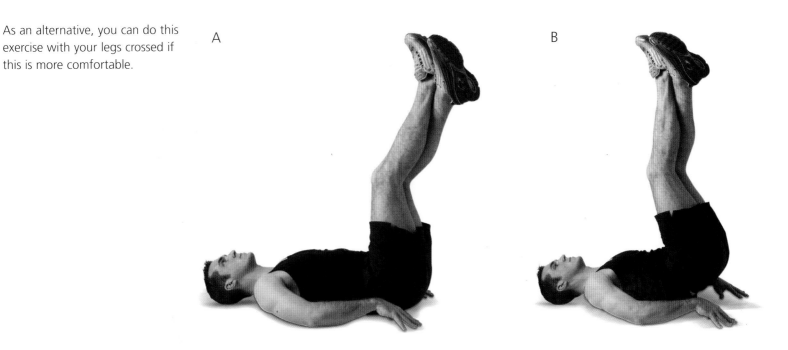

Exercise 12: leg raises (no weight)

This exercise works both your upper and lower abs.

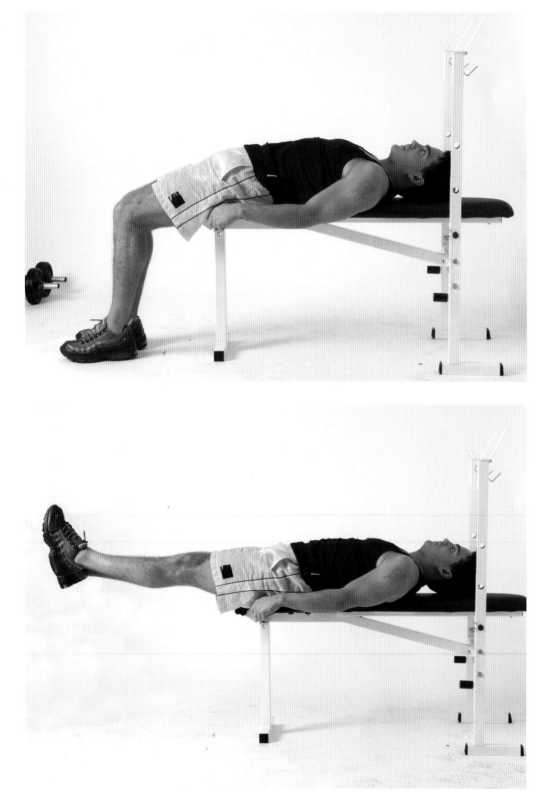

A Lie on your back on a bench, with your hips close to the edge. Grasp the corners of the bench near to your hips and extend your legs straight outwards, with your toes pointed.

B Keeping your legs together (don't lock your knees), slowly raise them to a vertical position. Hold the position for a second, then lower your legs, using a controlled motion, until your body is completely horizontal. Hold for a second and then lower your feet to the floor.

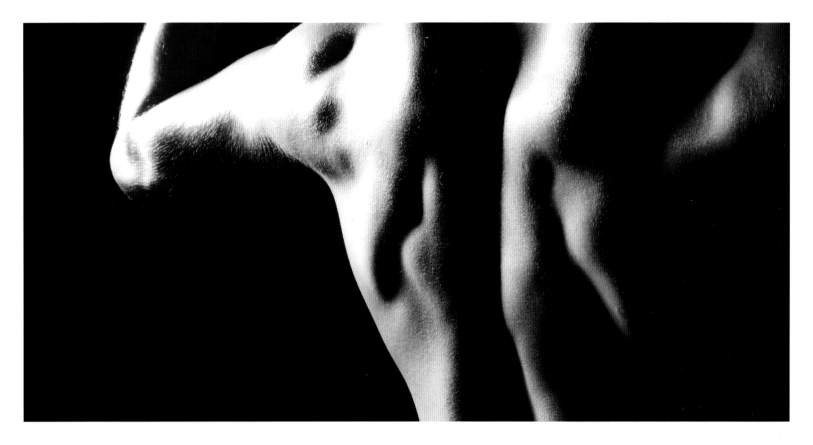

How to gain a powerful back

Many people forget about exercising their backs, probably because they can't see them. And, let's face it, the muscles of the back do not provide such an obviously powerful, sculpted look as the muscles of the chest (although well-defined back muscles do contribute to the desirable 'V'-shaped look that we would all like to attain). This does not, however, mean that they are not as important as the muscles in the rest of your torso.

The muscles of your back support you and provide balance and stability. Taking care of your back muscles is vital if you are to perform every upper-body exercise, and many lower-body exercises, too. But be warned that it is very easy to injure this delicate portion of your body during exercise routines. This is why it is so important not to neglect this area, but to build it up carefully to withstand the stresses and strains that your exercise regimes demand of it.

Your back muscles allow you to pull really hard in every exercise, making a strong back extremely beneficial in terms of weight-training, also providing considerable health advantages as you undergo the inevitable ageing process.

The muscles of the back

The biggest muscle in the back is the latissimus dorsi (usually abbreviated to the lats). The lats extends from behind each armpit to the middle of the back, enabling you to pull your arms towards your body and contributing to the much-admired 'V' shape. In addition to the lats, other important muscular groups are the rhomboids and trapezius (see page 17). Developing these, together with the lats, will add to the definition and overall look of the back.

Exercise 1: Romanian dead-lift

This all-purpose exercise strengthens not only your back, but also your arms, shoulders and legs.

Caution

Use less weight than you would for a normal dead-lift (see page 95).

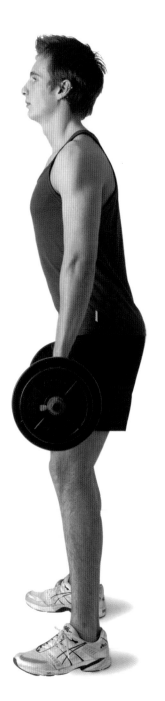

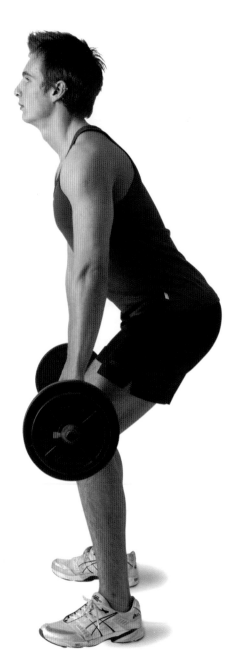

A Hold a lightly weighted barbell at mid-thigh level, with your hands more than a shoulder-width apart and your palms facing your body. Keep the barbell against your legs, with your arms fully extended, your back straight, your shoulders back and your chest pushed out. Pause for a second.

B Slowly bend forward at the hips, keeping the barbell close to your thighs. Your back should remain straight and your knees should be slightly bent. Slowly lower the barbell towards the floor as far as you comfortably can. Using a slow, controlled movement, and keeping your back straight, return to the starting position.

Exercise 2: wide-grip row

This versatile move also works your back deltoids, bottom and abs.

A Stand with your feet a shoulder-width apart and your knees slightly bent. Without arching your back, bend forward at the waist until your upper body is parallel with the floor. Grab a barbell using a grip wider than shoulder-width, with your palms facing your body.

B Raise the barbell during a count of two until it touches your chest. Your elbows should be higher than your back. Hold the position for a second, then slowly lower the barbell to about the middle of your shins.

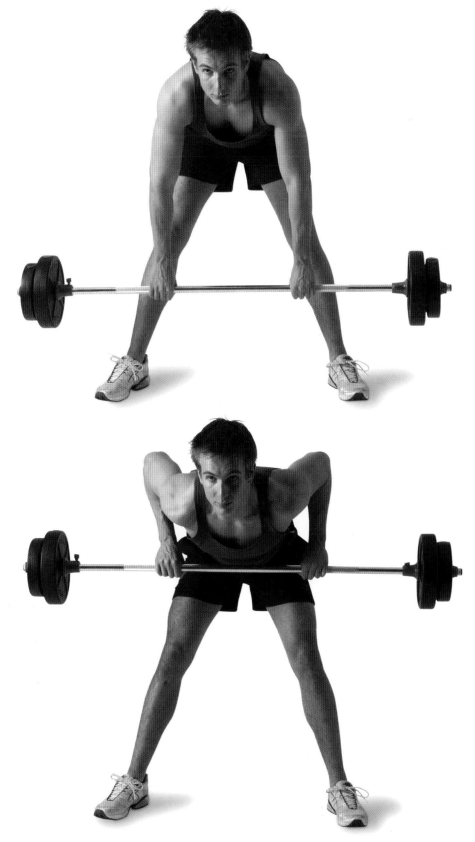

Exercise 3: one-arm dumbbell row

This movement also works your trapezius muscles, part of the shoulders.

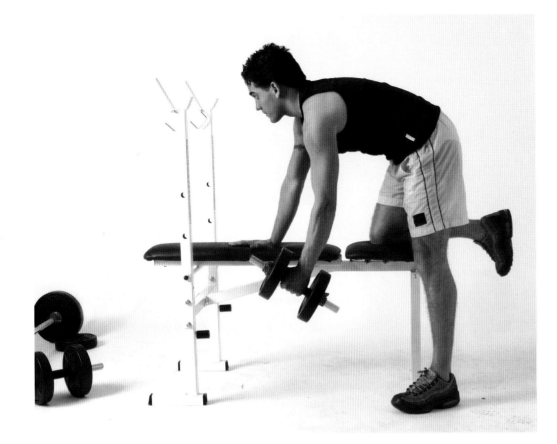

A   With a dumbbell in your left hand, rest your right knee and right hand on the centre line of a bench. Place your left foot firmly on the floor, with your knee slightly bent. Keep your back straight and your eyes facing downwards. Let your left arm hang down (don't lock your elbow), with your palm facing your left side.

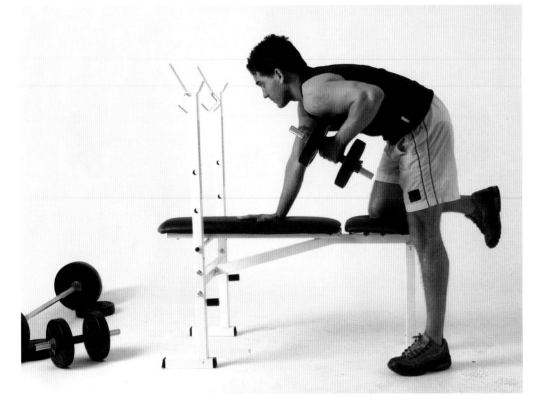

B   Slowly pull the dumbbell upwards and inwards, toward your torso, raising it as high as you can towards your chest. Your left elbow should point upwards, towards the ceiling, as you lift. Hold the position for a second, then return to the starting position.

Finish the set, then switch to your right side and repeat the exercise.

Exercise 4: toe touch

This exercise will strengthen your gluteal muscles and hamstrings.

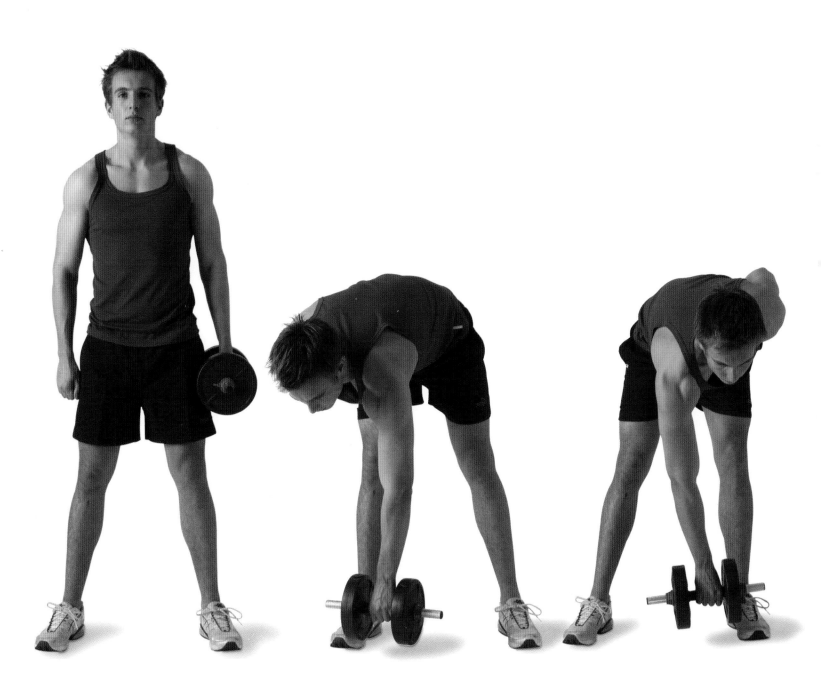

A Hold a dumbbell in your left hand, with your feet a shoulder-width apart and your knees unlocked.

B Slowly bend forwards, and to the right, and touch the dumbbell against your right foot. Hold the position for a second, then slowly return to the starting position.

C Finish the set, then switch sides and repeat the exercise.

Exercise 5: dumbbell swing

This move, which is great for strengthening your lower back, also strengthens your hamstrings, deltoids and glutes. Unlike most weight exercises, it should be done using an explosive movement.

Caution
Start by using very light weights and performing high repetitions.

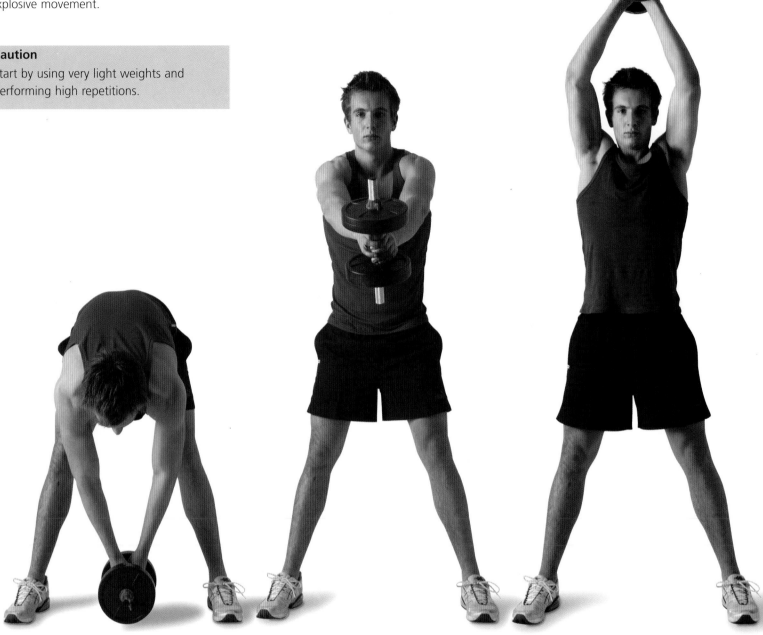

A   Holding a dumbbell in both hands, stand with your feet more than a shoulder-width apart and your knees unlocked. Bend forward at the waist until you are holding the dumbbell between your shins, with your arms fully extended and your back straight. (Keep the weight off the floor.)

B   Swing the dumbbell until it is over your head and you are standing upright, with your back still held straight.

C   Hold the dumbbell over your head for a second, then bend at the waist as you return to the starting position.

Exercise 6: dead-lift

This versatile move also strengthens your legs, shoulders and arms.

A Stand upright, with a lightly weighted barbell in front of you. Keeping your back straight, bend over the barbell and grasp it with your hands, which should be a shoulder-width apart, palms facing downwards. Keep your legs stiff and fairly straight, but do not lock your knees. Keep your arms straight and do not lock your elbows.

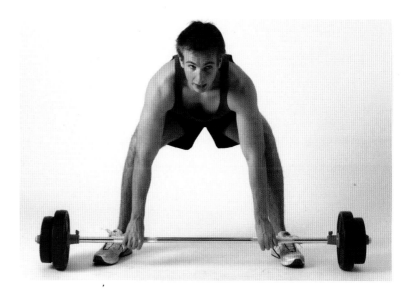

B Slowly lift the barbell to upper-thigh level. Your back, arms and legs should remain straight and your knees should not be locked. Hold the position for a second, then slowly lower the weight.

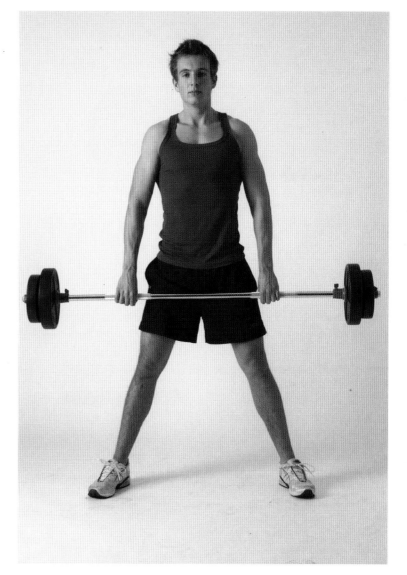

Exercise 7: chin-up

You will need a chin bar for this exercise, which also works your arms and shoulders.

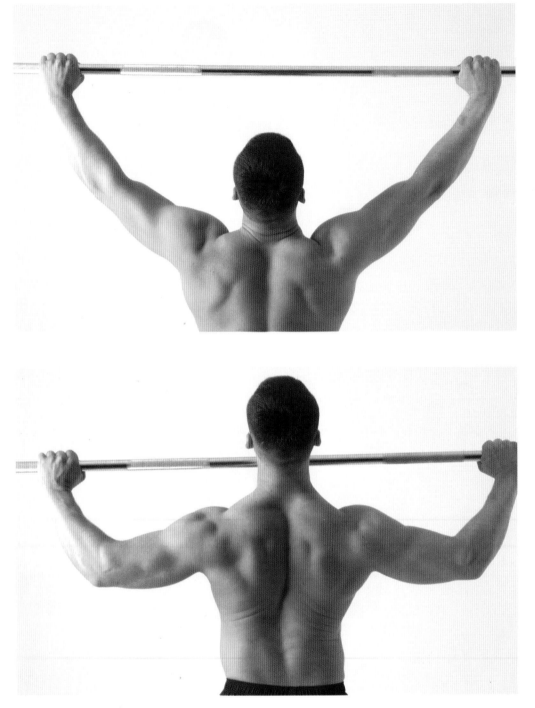

A   Suspend a handle from the chin bar and grasp it with both hands, so that you are hanging from the bar. Your knees should be slightly bent and your feet should be about 15cm (6in) above the floor when your arms are fully extended.

B   Slowly pull yourself up, using your lat muscles and not your biceps, until your torso almost touches your hands. Then slowly lower yourself down again.

Exercise 8: good morning

This move strengthens your lower back especially, and also works your hamstrings, abs and glutes. But it's difficult, and not recommended for beginners. To avoid injury, use an empty bar at first, and pay close attention to your form. Then move on to light weights until you have mastered the movement.

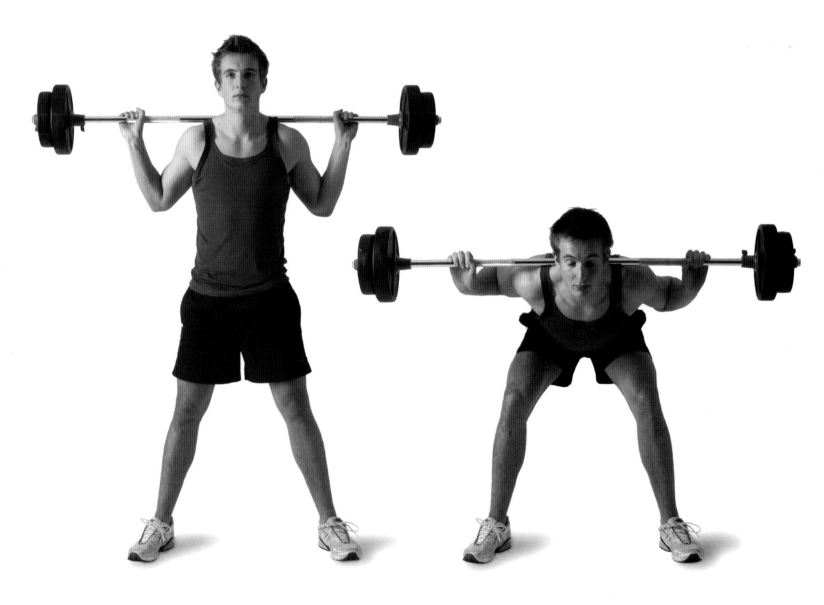

A Stand with your legs a shoulder-width apart, and don't lock your knees. Hold a barbell across your shoulders, with your hands slightly more than a shoulder-width apart and your palms facing outwards. Keep your upper body straight, your shoulders back and your chest pushed out as you lean forward slightly at the waist.

B Bend down slowly at the waist, keeping your back straight, until your upper body is parallel with the floor. You should be looking forward, not down. Hold the position for a second, then slowly return to the starting position.

Building powerful thighs

The thigh muscles are very obvious, being among the largest in the body. They are used in almost everything that we do, including walking, running, climbing and, indeed, all sports. Yet the muscles of the legs are often ignored in weight-training by trainers who are intent on working their upper bodies alone. You should, however, spend as much time on, and pay as much attention to, the muscles of your legs as you would to those of your upper body because neglecting these important muscle groups will inevitably result in an off-balanced look.

Leg exercises admittedly take up a lot of effort and energy, but in my opinion they also constitute good overall body-building exercises, making them well worth the time and trouble. Combine proper nutrition with good-quality exercise, and you'll achieve powerful legs.

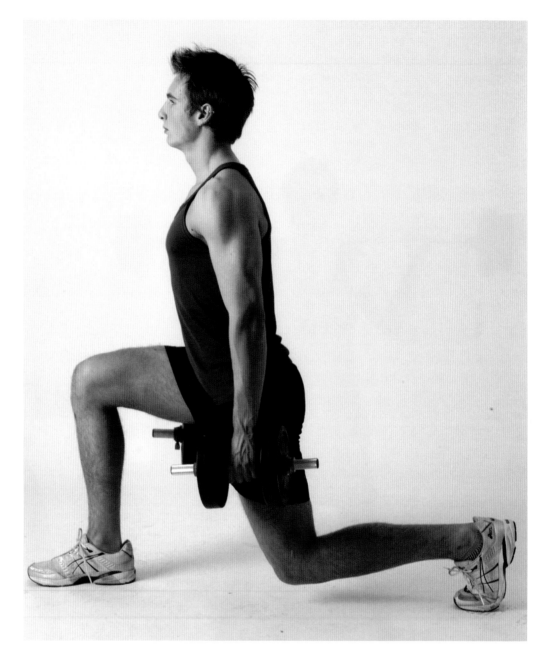

The muscles of the thighs

The quadrilaterals, or 'quads', are a group of four large muscles in the upper legs that allow you to extend your knees and your thighs at the hip. The hamstrings, comprising three muscle groups at the back of your thighs, run from the knees to the hip and allow you to bend your knees.

The quads should be stronger than the hamstrings, although the hamstrings should not be neglected. The literal meaning of the word 'hamstring' is 'to render powerless', and because this group of muscles is a weak point, it's important to take great care to maintain the correct balance when working the two muscle groups.

Exercise 1: Drop squat

This great all-purpose exercise conditions large muscle groups (specifically your thighs and gluteal muscles), while also working your shoulders, back, arms and legs.

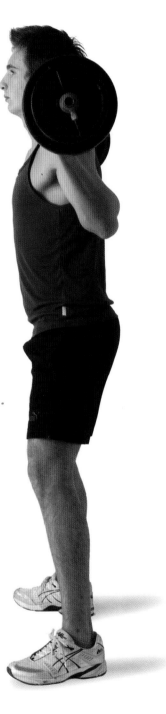

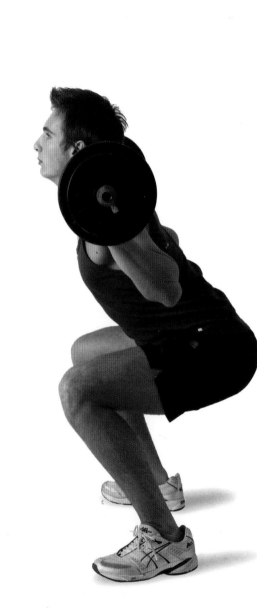

A Place a barbell evenly across your upper back and shoulders. Stand up straight, with your feet a shoulder-width apart and your toes pointing slightly outwards. Don't drop your head, which should be in line with your torso, with your eyes looking ahead.

B Keeping your feet flat and torso straight, slightly bend your knees and slowly squat down. Don't arch your back or let your knees extend far beyond your toes. Squat until your thighs are almost parallel with the floor. Pause, then slowly rise to the starting position.

Exercise 2: hack squat

This variation of the squat puts less pressure on your knees and lower back than the normal squat (see Exercise 1), but requires greater balancing skills.

Caution

To avoid injury, start with an unweighted barbell, then slowly add more weight as you master the movement. (You should still use less weight than you would for a normal squat.)

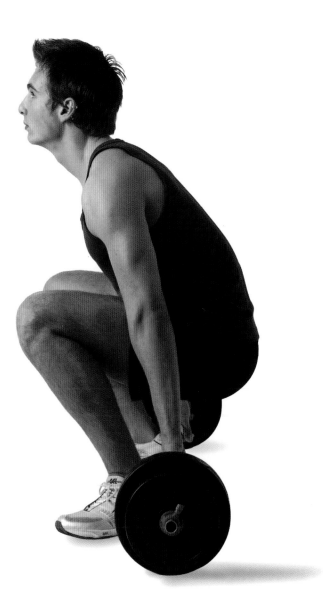

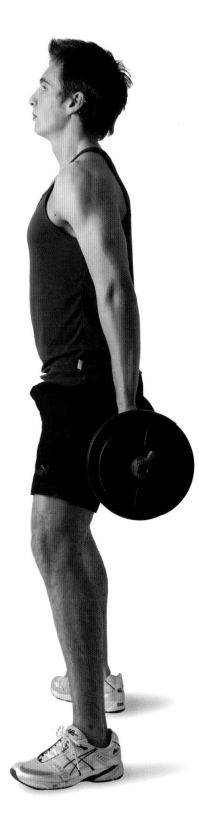

A Stand with your feet a shoulder-width apart, with a barbell positioned directly behind your heels. Squat down and grip the bar, with your palms facing away from your body.

B Your hands should be slightly more than a shoulder-width apart. Now stand up, holding the bar at arm's length behind your thighs. Keep your head in line with your body.

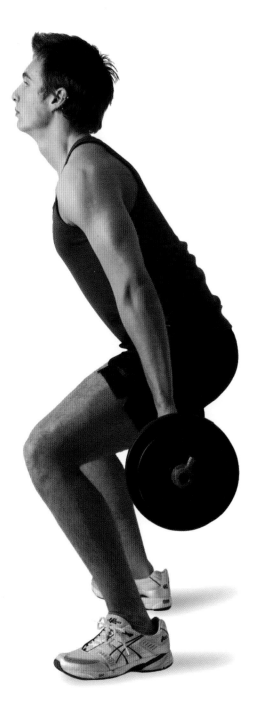

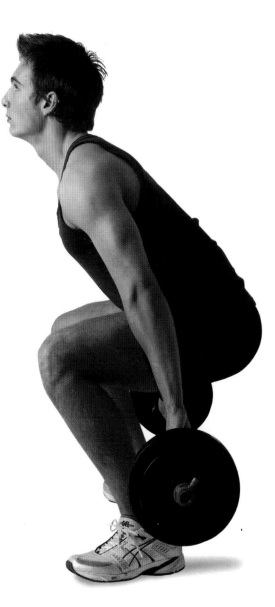

C   Slowly squat down until your thighs are nearly parallel with the floor.

D   Hold the position for a second, then slowly rise, keeping your arms fully extended.

Exercise 3: dumbbell power lunge

This advanced exercise also works your gluteal and hamstring muscles. Use light weights to start with.

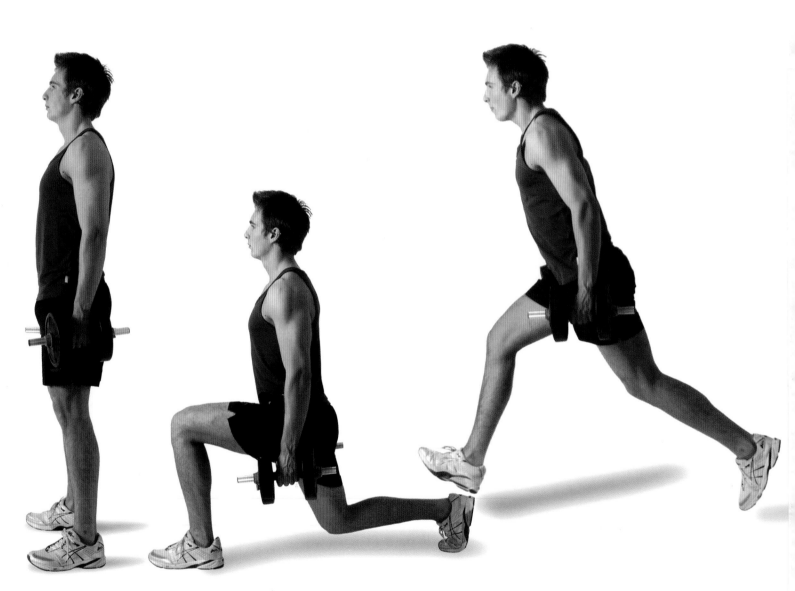

A   Stand upright, holding a dumbbell firmly in each hand. Your arms should be fully extended by your sides, with your palms facing inwards. Your feet should be about a hip-width apart and your torso should be upright, although you should maintain a natural curve in your lower back.

B   Using your left leg, step forward slightly further than you would when taking a normal step. Keep your upper body upright, with your arms by your sides and the dumbbells positioned roughly in line with the centre of your body. Bend your left leg to an angle of 90° (you should still be able to see your toes when looking down). Bend your right leg slightly at the knee. (Your right heel will rise a little, but your foot should remain in the same position.)

C   Now explosively jump upwards, switching legs in mid-air so that your right leg is forward and your left leg is back on landing. That's one rep. As soon as you land, push off and switch legs again.

Exercise 4: leg extension with ankle weights

Using different foot positions can change how the muscles are worked in this movement. Try pointing your toes backwards or straight forwards to work different parts of your quads.

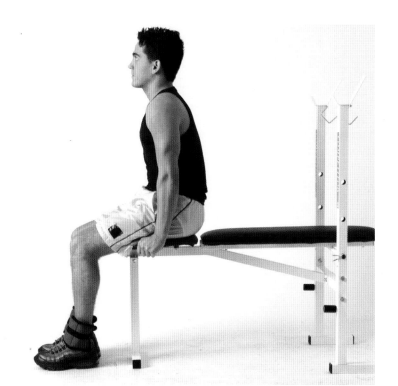

A Fasten ankle weights around your ankles. Sit on a bench, grasping its sides with your hands. Your knees should be bent at an angle of 90° or slightly more, and your toes should be pointing forwards.

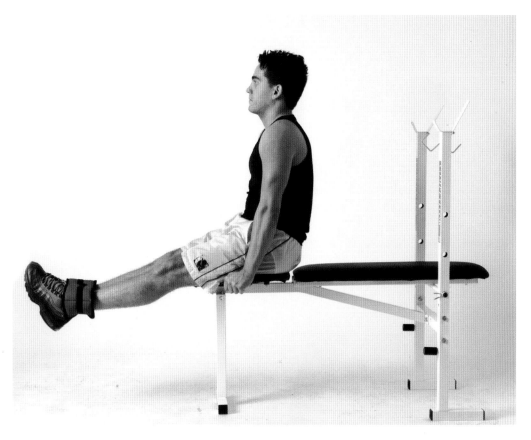

B Using the sides of the bench for support, slowly straighten your legs by lifting your ankles and contracting your quadriceps. Don't lock your knees at full extension. Your toes should be pointing upwards and outwards at an angle of about 45° to the floor. Hold the position for a second, then slowly lower your legs to the starting position.

Exercise 5: lateral squat

This exercise works your gluteal muscles, as well as the sides of your thighs. If you are a beginner, you could use dumbbells instead of a barbell.

A   Stand up straight and grip a barbell positioned evenly across your upper back and shoulders, with your hands slightly more than a shoulder-width apart and your palms facing away from your body. Place your feet in a wide stance, with your toes pointing outwards, and keep your head in line with your body.

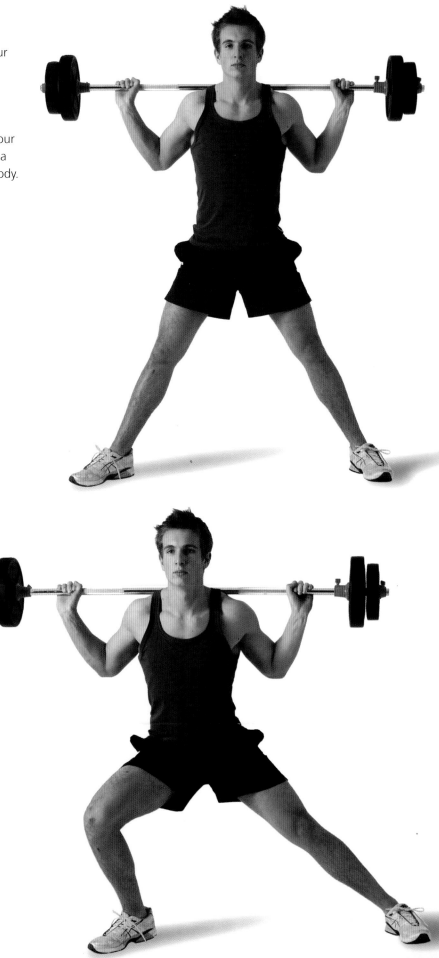

B   Drop down by slowly bending your right leg until your right thigh is parallel with the floor. Don't let your right knee turn inwards or extend beyond your toes. Put most of your weight on your right leg, keeping your left leg extended, with the knee slightly bent. Hold this stance for a second, then return to the starting position by slowly extending your right leg and bringing your torso back to the centre.

Without resting, repeat the exercise using your left leg. That makes one repetition.

Exercise 6: leg curl with ankle weights

This exercise also works the erector spinae muscles of your lower back.

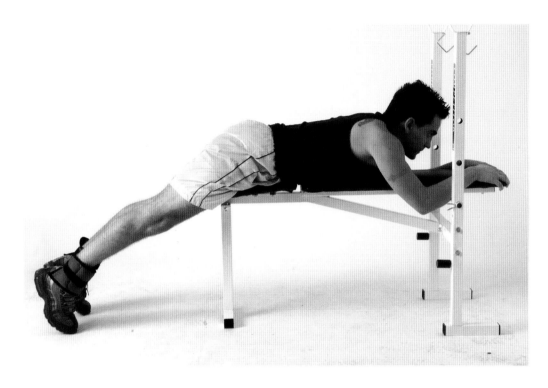

A Secure an ankle weight to each ankle. Now lie on your stomach on a bench, with both legs extending straight outwards. Your knees should extend just beyond the edge of the bench, enabling you to bend your legs upwards. If necessary, hold on to the legs of the bench for support.

B Keeping your feet together and pointing outwards, slowly curl the weights towards your bottom, using a semi-circular motion, until your legs are at an angle of about 90°. Point your toes upwards, but don't arch your pelvis or back. Your body should remain flush with the bench. Hold the position for a second, then slowly lower your legs to the starting position.

Exercise 7: double-leg squat jump

This exercise also works your bottom muscles and hamstrings.

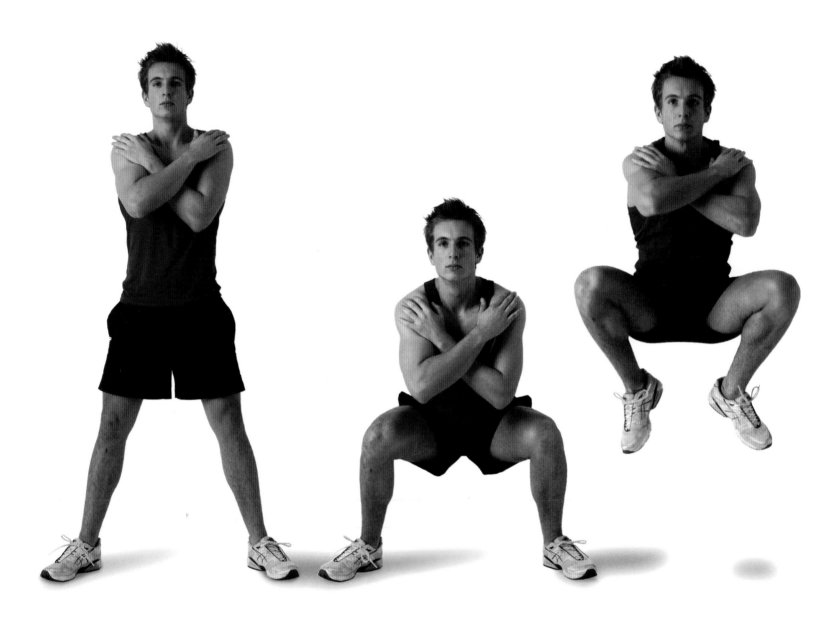

A Stand with your feet slightly more than a shoulder-width apart and your arms crossed in front of you.

B Keeping your head up and your back straight, squat until your thighs are almost parallel with the floor.

C Jump straight upwards, using an explosive movement. Don't let your lower legs provide all of the power, but instead make your bottom, thighs and hips work. As soon as you land, squat and jump again without resting.

Exercise 8: single-leg squat

This exercise also strengthens your gluteal muscles, hips and back.

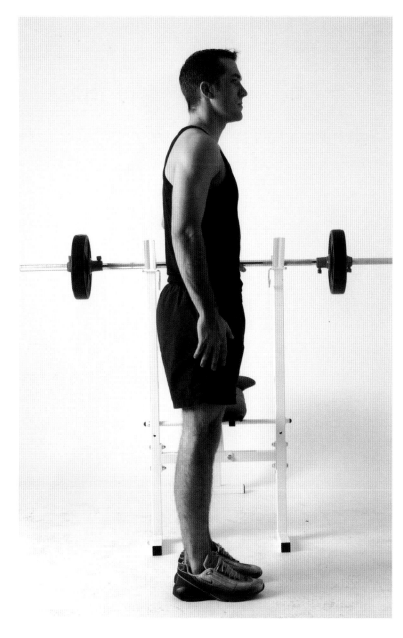 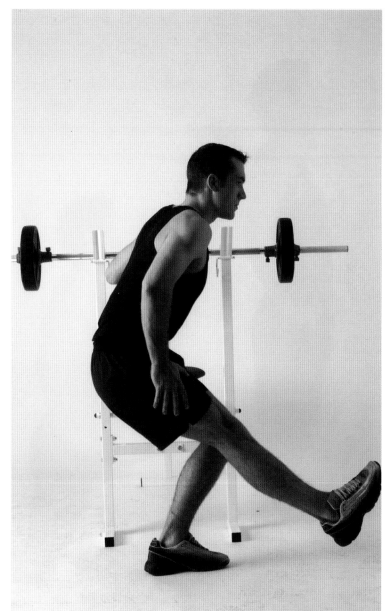

A   Position a sturdy chair or piece of exercise equipment to your left so that you can rest your left hand on it for balance. Stand upright, with your feet a shoulder-width apart and your knees slightly bent. Keep your back straight and put your right hand on your hip for balance.

B   Keeping your back straight, slowly begin to squat on your left leg while extending your right leg in front of you. As soon as your left thigh is parallel with the floor, slowly press yourself back up into the starting position. Don't pause between repetitions – you should look like a piston pumping up and down.

Finish the set, then switch legs and repeat the exercise.

Exercise 9: alternating jump lunge

This explosive move also works your gluteal muscles.

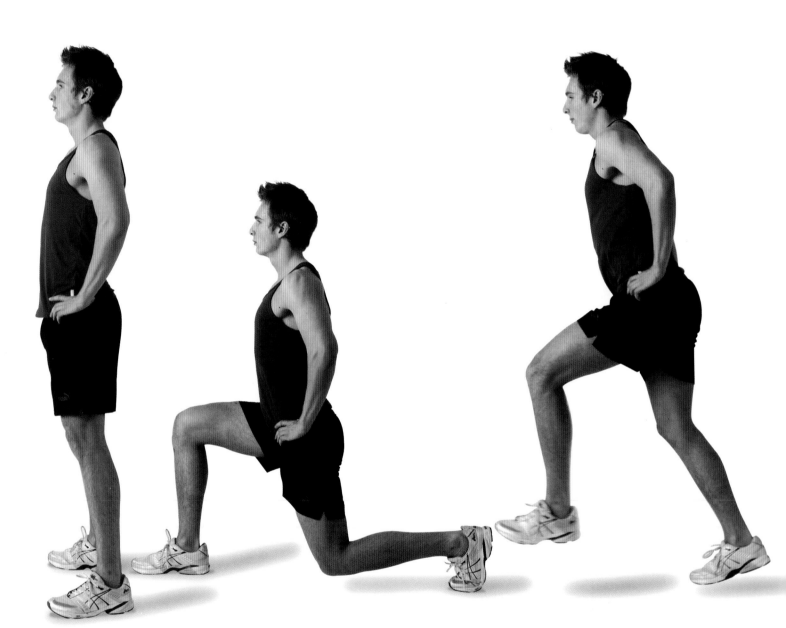

A   Stand with your feet a shoulder-width apart and your back straight.

B   Take a long step forward with your right foot. Firmly plant that foot on the floor and bend your knee until your right thigh is parallel with the floor. Don't let your right knee extend beyond your right foot. Your left leg should be extended behind you, the knee slightly bent and the heel raised. Keep your upper body upright and your head in line with your spine.

C   Now quickly and explosively push off on your right foot, extending your left leg in front of you. You should end up in much the same lunging position as before, but with your left foot in front of you and your right foot behind you. Immediately push off on your left foot, extending your right leg forward again. That's one repetition.

Repeat without resting until you've finished the set.

Exercise 10: phantom chair

This exercise also works your gluteal muscles.

A   Stand leaning against a wall, with your back flat against it and
    your knees slightly bent. Your feet should be positioned a little
    more than a shoulder-width apart, about 50cm (1ft) away from
    the wall, and your toes should be pointing slightly outwards.
    Keep your shoulders back and your chest pushed out.

B   Slowly bend your knees, lowering yourself until the tops of your
    thighs are parallel with the ground, but don't go so far that your
    knees extend beyond your toes. Hold the position until your
    muscles are fatigued, then slowly straighten your legs and return
    to the starting position.

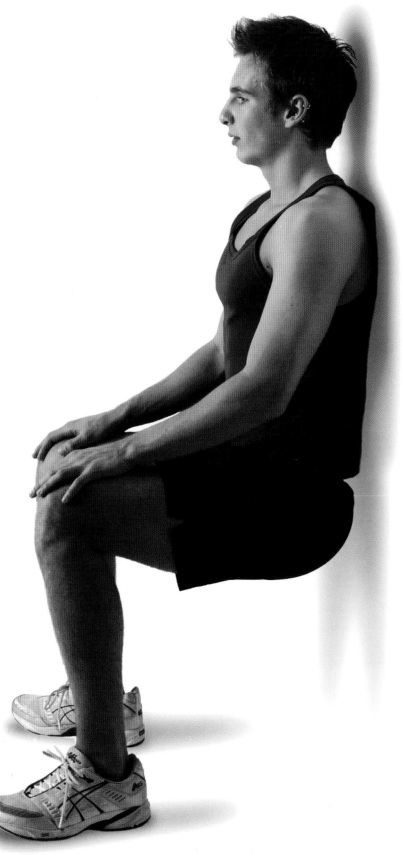

A word about calf muscles

Exercising your thigh muscles will also cause your calves to develop. A simple and perfect exercise for further developing your calf muscles is as follows.

Calf raises

You will need a platform of some kind for this simple exercise. A large, sturdy book about 5 to 8cm (2 to 3in) thick would be suitable.

> **Caution**
> All exercise requires great care, but move C in particular must be performed very carefully indeed.

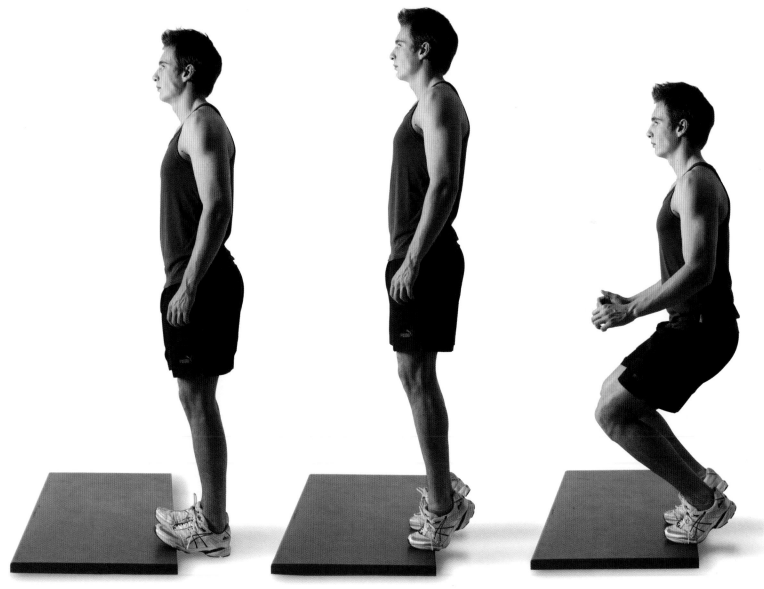

A   Stand with your heels placed firmly on the floor and the balls of your feet slightly elevated on your platform. Your toes should be pointing upwards a little.

B   Slowly raise your body by placing your weight on the balls of your feet and lifting your heels from the floor until you feel your calf muscles pulling. Hold this position for a second and then slowly lower yourself to the starting position.

Begin with ten repetitions of this move, slowly building up the number of repetitions as your weight-training regime progresses.

C   Slowly bend your elbows to an angle of 90° while simultaneously lowering your bottom towards the floor and raising your heels. Now push yourself back down to the starting position.

Index

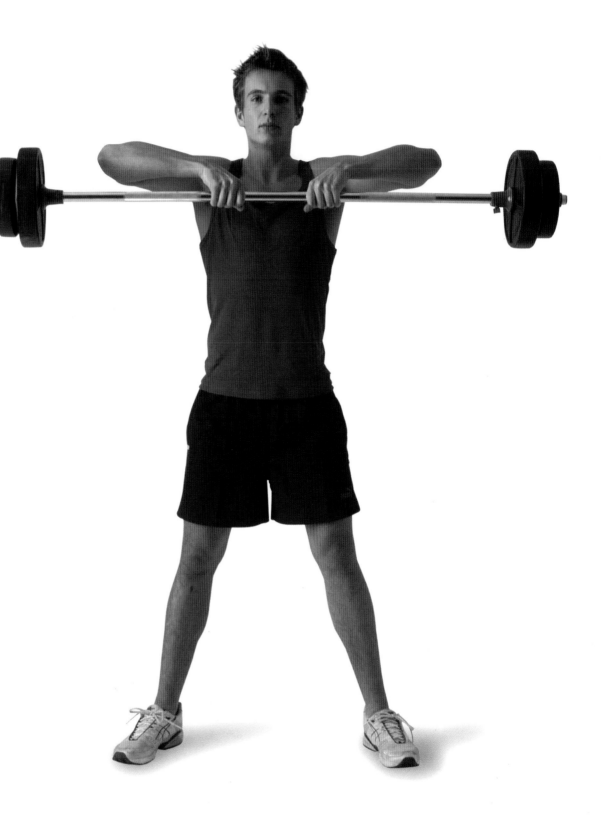

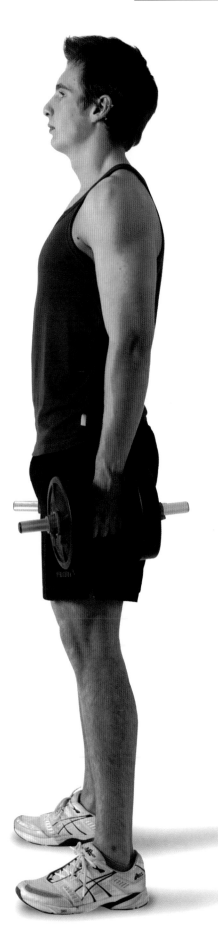

Credits

I would like to thank Jon Dee for being so kind and helpful all the years I've known him.

Acknowledgements

The author and publishers would like to thank Russell Myers, Luke Pomaro and Adam Whilding for being models in this book.

Images pp 12t, 12bl, 14-16, 21, 22bl, 23bl, 24, 26m, 26b, 35-39 © Getty Images

Images pp 25, 26t, 27-34, 38tl © Stockbyte

(where b = bottom, m = middle, t = top, l = left)